Beyond Transference

When the Therapist's Real Life Intrudes

Beyond Transference

When the Therapist's Real Life Intrudes

Edited by
Judith H. Gold, M.D., F.R.C.P.C.
John C. Nemiah, M.D.

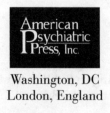

American
Psychiatric
Press, Inc.

Washington, DC
London, England

Note: The authors have worked to ensure that all information in this book concerning drug dosages, schedules, and routes of administration is accurate as of the time of publication and consistent with standards set by the U.S. Food and Drug Administration and the general medical community. As medical research and practice advance, however, therapeutic standards may change. For this reason and because human and mechanical errors sometimes occur, we recommend that readers follow the advice of a physician who is directly involved in their care or the care of a member of their family.

Copyright © 1993 American Psychiatric Press, Inc.
ALL RIGHTS RESERVED
Manufactured in the United States of America on acid-free paper
96 95 94 93 4 3 2 1

First Edition
American Psychiatric Press, Inc.
1400 K Street, N.W., Washington, DC 20005

Library of Congress Cataloging-in-Publication Data
Beyond transference : when the therapist's real life intrudes / edited
  by Judith H. Gold, John C. Nemiah. — 1st ed.
      p.   cm.
  Includes bibliographical references and index.
  ISBN 0-88048-361-X
  1. Transference (Psychology) 2. Psychotherapist and patient.
  3. Countertransference (Psychology)   I. Gold, Judith H., 1941–   .
  II. Nemiah, John C. (John Case), 1918–   .
  [DNLM: 1. Countertransference (Psychology) 2. Professional
  -Patient Relations. 3. Psychotherapy. MW 62 B573]
  RC489.T73B49 1993
  616.89'14—dc20
  DNLM/DLC   92-7053
  for Library of Congress   CIP

British Library Cataloguing in Publication Data
A CIP record is available from the British Library.

Contents

Contributors

Stephen J. Bartels, M.D.
Assistant Clinical Professor of Psychiatry, Dartmouth Medical
School; Medical Director, West Central Community Mental Health
Services, Hanover, New Hampshire

Harry Beskind, M.D.
Adjunct Professor of Psychiatry, Dartmouth Medical School; Private
practice in psychiatry and psychoanalysis, Norwich, Vermont

Mollie Brooks, M.S.W.
Private practice in psychoanalytic psychotherapy, Norwich, Vermont

Richard B. Ferrell, M.D.
Associate Professor of Clinical Psychiatry, Department of Psychiatry,
Dartmouth Medical School, Hanover, New Hampshire

Judith H. Gold, M.D., F.R.C.P.C.
Private practice in psychiatry, Halifax, Nova Scotia, Canada

Henry Grunebaum, M.D.
Director, Family Studies, Harvard Medical School, Department of
Psychiatry, Cambridge Hospital, Cambridge, Massachusetts

Keith H. Johansen, M.D.
Clinical Professor of Psychiatry, Southwestern Medical School,
University of Texas, Dallas, Texas

Alex H. Kaplan, M.D.
Clinical Professor of Psychiatry, Washington University; Faculty,
St. Louis Psychoanalytic Institute, St. Louis, Missouri

Carol C. Nadelson, M.D.
Professor and Associate Chair, Department of Psychiatry, Tufts
University School of Medicine, New England Medical Hospitals,
Boston, Massachusetts

John C. Nemiah, M.D.
Professor of Psychiatry Emeritus, Harvard Medical School; Professor
of Psychiatry, Dartmouth Medical School, Hanover, New Hampshire

Malkah T. Notman, M.D.
Clinical Professor of Psychiatry, Harvard Medical School; Acting
Chairperson, Department of Psychiatry, The Cambridge Hospital,
Cambridge, Massachusetts

Trevor R. P. Price, M.D.
Professor and Chairman, Department of Psychiatry, Allegheny
Campus, Medical College of Pennsylvania, Pittsburgh, Pennsylvania

James M. Trench, M.D.
Lecturer in Psychiatry, Yale University School of Medicine, Mystic,
Connecticut

Maureen Sayers Van Niel, M.D.
Instructor, Harvard Medical School; Attending Psychiatrist, Brigham
and Women's Hospital, Boston, Massachusetts

Introduction

The various and numerous issues that affect the lives of everyone also affect the life and, potentially, the functioning of the therapist. Although many patients at some time see their therapist as omnipotent and, therefore, problem free, this is only a vision colored by transference and, unfortunately, not an accurate perception. Real-life events occur for us all, and the chapters in this volume demonstrate that therapists are not immune to their effects, nor often is the therapy. The importance of that influence on the conduct and content of the therapeutic process must not be forgotten or diminished. Psychotherapy deals with the interactions between people and within persons, exemplified by the therapeutic relationship. Overlooking the effects on the therapist of events in his or her own life will interfere with and hinder the work necessary to bring therapy to a successful conclusion.

Some events in the personal life of a therapist are very obvious, such as a pregnancy, absence due to illness, or changes in an office or in office personnel. Some are obvious because the daily lives of the therapist and patient mingle, whether through living in a small community, working in the same hospital, or having mutual friends or neighbors. These latter situations can occur in a town of any size and may be due to referral patterns as much as to chance meetings at a concert or while shopping. Other events may not be known to the patient, who may still sense a discomfort or change in the therapist and without knowing the true cause may ascribe the change to something they imagine they have said or done in the therapy session. As pointed out in the chapters that follow, the therapist must be aware of these possibilities and be prepared to deal with them so that the patient's personalization of the therapist's behavior is acknowledged and the situation is clarified and, if necessary, corrected.

For example, an anxious woman with very low self-esteem due to a long history of abuse and neglect reported with much affect that she had dreamt the reason her regular appointment had been canceled one week was because the therapist was "taking a trip to another city to have your hair done. You agreed to meet me for a few minutes at the airport but you walked right by me. I woke up so angry at you." Despite having had the absence explained in advance, this young woman could not believe that anyone would find her worthwhile enough to treat, but also felt that her suffering was not being acknowledged once again.

The patient who has survived abuse is especially likely to interpret all actions of the therapist personally, based on a multifaceted set of psychodynamics, and constantly requires reassurances in deed and words that the therapist cares when no else has. This situation is made infinitely more complex if the patient was sexually abused by a previous therapist or if a history of childhood abuse was minimized in previous therapy.

Because we are more cognizant now of the actual prevalence of incest among our patients, the origins and significance of certain behaviors in therapy have become clearer than they were before incest was recognized as an unfortunately rather common event. The therapist must be mindful of the often exquisite sensitivity to inattention or oversight in such patients. Additionally, these people are often abused again in future relationships. We are only beginning to acknowledge, discuss, and censure colleagues who abuse their patients and to believe patients' reports of such behavior. In Chapter 9, Malkah Notman deals with this neglected topic, one that many in the field would prefer to ignore. Gaining the trust of individuals who have been abused, as children or as adults, is a delicate task that arouses a mixture of reactions in the therapist. Again, the sensitivity of such people to the actions, words, and affect of the therapist can be exquisite.

At times, the therapist must take the initiative and explain even an obvious situation briefly so the session can proceed as usual. An example of such an event was the flooding of a therapist's office by a faulty air-conditioning system over a weekend. Patients were seen amidst torn-up carpeting and scattered furniture and books. Some appointments had to be rescheduled. A concise but calm statement about what had happened precluded the formation of erroneous assumptions so that the therapist was able to devote the usual attention to the patient without seeming distracted.

Most patients are curious about their therapist and the facts of the therapist's life. Some ask, some imagine details, some find answers through daily contacts at work or in social situations. Often training of residents does not include discussions of how to deal with these instances that occur outside of the office. How should you react to finding a patient in your aerobics class or teaching your child?

We have asked the authors to address these real-life events based on their own experiences and knowledge of those of their colleagues. Sharing their feelings with the reader in such a personal format reflects the theme of the book: current issues in transference and countertransference. Here and throughout the book, the term *countertransference* is used to include, as stated in Chapter 5 by Keith Johansen, "all of the emotional reactions of the therapist toward the patient." Life events can leave the therapist with a mixture of emotions that at times may be similar to those of some of his or her patients. Also, listening to the patient may arouse, consciously or unconsciously, feelings within the therapist that can interfere with treatment. In each chapter, despite the divergence of topics, certain themes are repeated. The reactions of the therapist are comparative whether coping with illness, the illness of a loved one, divorce, a malpractice suit, or pregnancy. In all of these events the therapist acts in response to the uncertainty of changing personal circumstances.

Absences also must be dealt with, both emotionally and rationally, not only in terms of the patient's response but also in practice management. One can return from holiday or a conference to a pile of messages and paperwork. If this frazzles the therapist, less attention will be paid to the patient and the nuances of therapy, and this inattention will magnify any negative feelings the patient already has about the break in treatment. In Chapter 4, Carol Nadelson writes about her own experiences as a busy therapist who has frequent absences due to other professional commitments and details the responses and insights of other similar therapists.

Therapists are accustomed to lending ego strength to their patients as the individuals learn to develop their own ego resources. When the "healer" requires all that strength personally, the therapy and the patient suffer. We pass on to our patients a sense of personal mastery and control over one's life as well as hope for the future and trust in others. The shaken and preoccupied therapist cannot do this or properly assist the patient. These points are discussed thoroughly in Chapter 2 by Harry Grunebaum and Chapter 3 by Alex Kaplan. It may be difficult at times like these for a therapist to find someone with whom to discuss personal situations or countertransference problems. In a small community it may be impossible, or seem to be impossible. The role of supervision is highlighted in such circumstances in a number of the chapters and discussed more fully by James Trench in Chapter 6.

Absences can also be used as an opportunity for consultation and exchange with colleagues when supervision on a regular basis is unobtainable at home. Although obviously not preferable to regular supervision, at times these interactions can be very useful, especially for the therapist who practices in a small or isolated community. Some problems may be more comfortably discussed away from home. The vulnerability felt during the divorce process may be one of these instances, whereas working through feelings around illness and the loss of a spouse may be more readily dealt with locally.

The therapist who is struggling with personal events may turn to work with patients as a coping mechanism. This theme is also repeated in several of the chapters. Returning to work too quickly after illness or loss can be a defensive maneuver but may not allow the therapist to appreciate or interpret properly what the patient is saying and feeling. Trying to ignore or deny one's own feelings is often unsuccessful and may be confusing to the patient. Further, countertransference responses can lead to misinterpretation of the patient's words and actions and to inappropriate suggestions to and management of patients. Patients may feel that they have to help the therapist. It is important for the therapist to recognize and consider the meaning of their real event to the particular patient and how this can affect the working through of previous traumas for that individual.

Psychiatry has undergone many changes in the last two decades. With the growth of psychopharmacotherapy and the varieties of psychotherapy available, we have moved away from the passive stance of classic psychoanalysis and psychodynamic psychotherapy. Our patients are less willing to accept the authority of any caregiver unquestioningly and demand to know about all aspects of their treatment, including the personal life of their therapist. The therapist must be more flexible in the use of treatments and more willing to self-disclose than in earlier years. It is more important than ever that a therapist has good insight and remains aware of countertransference reactions and feelings during sessions with patients. Furthermore, we are learning that there are many aspects to the etiologies of psychopathology, as well as to treatment modalities, including the therapist's life events and personality. Countertransference issues have always been discussed and known to be important to the conduct and outcome of therapy. In this book we look beyond the intrapsychic to those very real events that affect the therapist and thus the therapeutic interaction itself.

Judith H. Gold, M.D., F.R.C.P.C.

Chapter 1

Practical and Theoretical Dilemmas of Dynamic Psychotherapy in a Small Community

Harry Beskind, M.D.
Stephen J. Bartels, M.D.
Mollie Brooks, M.S.W.

Traditional models of psycho-therapeutic technique assume that a clear separation between the personal and professional roles of the therapist and patient is essential to proper and effective treatment. The urban environment in which most psychotherapists train and practice provides a setting in which a therapist's personal life can easily remain private, and contacts with patients outside of the office are rare or nonexistent. Yet for the dynamic psychotherapist who lives and practices in a small community, this clear separation is impossible to maintain. Instead, the small town practitioner is routinely challenged by personal and clinical situations unanticipated by traditional models of psychotherapeutic technique. In this chapter we describe the practical dilemmas of conducting dynamic psychotherapy in a small community and the implications for reexamining basic assumptions of dynamic theory.

A limited literature has reported some of the dilemmas confronting the psychotherapist in a small town setting. In the small community, contacts with patients outside of the therapeutic hour are frequent and unavoidable. The therapist routinely runs into patients in public, social, and professional settings. The high visibility associated with being a professional in the community may result in loss of privacy and lack of anonymity (Copans and Racusin 1983; Moffic 1981; Riggs and Kugel 1976). Paradoxically, social and professional isolation is commonly reported as a complication of rural practice (Hargrove 1982; Jeffrey and Reeve 1978; Van Dyke 1986). For many therapists who have trained and practiced in an urban setting, the move to a rural area is made without

1

a full appreciation of the complexities of rural practice (Copans and Racusin 1983; Riggs and Kugel 1976). These personal and professional stresses are compounded by the realization that many assumptions inherent to traditional models of psychotherapy do not readily apply to the realities of rural practice (Hargrove 1986; Mazer 1976; Moffic 1981; Riggs and Kugel 1976).

In an attempt to further understand the experience of small town practice, 15 dynamically oriented therapists in the Upper Connecticut Valley of New Hampshire and Vermont were interviewed in an open format with specific attention to the impact of setting and community on personal and professional life. The reflections of these therapists are synthesized in this chapter with the goal of identifying traditional practices of dynamic therapists that are often put to a test in a small community. First, we describe the general differences in practice between urban and small communities. Next, we address four common problems in small town practice: 1) overlapping roles in the community, 2) confidentiality, 3) loss of anonymity, and 4) adjustment to practice in a small town. We illustrate these problems with case examples selected from our interviews (disguised to protect the confidentiality of patients and therapists). Finally, we conclude with a discussion of the practical and theoretical implications for the practice of psychotherapy.

CONTRAST IN THERAPY: URBAN VERSUS SMALL COMMUNITY SETTINGS

For the purpose of this chapter, we interviewed 15 therapists living and practicing in towns with populations of less than 5,000. We use the terms *small community* and *small town* interchangeably to mean a small, self-contained community characterized by a relative uniformity of population, traditional values with little diversity, and frequent interaction between many members of the community in different roles. In the small community there is little or no isolation of social systems. Not all small communities are rural; some suburban towns may share the characteristics of the small community. The small community stands in marked contrast to the urban setting, which is characterized by a large population and great social, economic, cultural, and professional diversity.

Urban settings automatically support a separation of the therapist's personal life from the daily lives of patients outside of the office. This separation facilitates one of the central elements of analytic psychotherapy: that the interaction between therapist and patient in the consultation room is a microcosm of what happens in the subjective world of the patient. Psychological material is analyzed and interpreted in a setting that is relatively constant and fully isolated from extratherapeutic contact.

In the small community setting, however, a clear division between personal lives and the professional therapeutic hour is usually impossible to maintain. It is common in small communities for a therapist to know people mentioned by patients during therapy sessions, including neighbors, friends, and colleagues of the therapist. Sometimes it is unavoidable for a therapist to treat people who know each other well. In these instances, the patient may be completely unaware of the therapist's independent knowledge of many intimate details of personal relationships. The therapist faces the difficulty of keeping the original sources of information straight and runs the risk of unintentionally disclosing confidential material.

The most evident and crucial difference between doing dynamic therapy in an urban setting as opposed to a small community is that therapists in the small community are constantly presented with the breakdown or potential confusion between the therapeutic alliance and the transference. The working alliance or real relationship (Greenson 1965; Greenson and Wexler 1969) or the therapeutic alliance (Sterba 1934) is stretched beyond the therapeutic hour. The "incestuousness" that is part of a small community makes it difficult to keep the boundaries of therapy from events outside the office. The idea that everything is "grist for the mill" in therapy is pushed to the limit and may push therapists beyond the limits they came to expect through urban training and practice.

PROBLEMS IN SMALL TOWN PRACTICE

Overlapping Roles in the Community

The overlapping of personal and professional roles is a characteristic and unavoidable aspect of living and working in a small community (Hargrove 1986). The child psychiatrist may have young patients who are classmates or friends of his or her own children. His or her children may share the same car pool, requiring that the therapist interact socially with the parents he or she also counsels. The therapist's spouse may be his or her patient's school teacher or may be a physician who treats members of the patient's family (Copans and Racusin 1983). Such crossovers happen frequently in small communities. Only if the therapist is not threatened transferentially will he or she be able to handle such overlapping of roles positively in the context of a dynamic understanding of the patient. The following case examples are typical of social encounters that every therapist sooner or later faces in a small community:

Case 1

A therapist and her patient, Ms. A, were close friends of the same person in town. When the friend's daughter was to be married, both the therapist and Ms. A were invited and were expected to attend the wedding. If the therapist declined the invitation, an important personal relationship would be threatened at a significant personal sacrifice for her. Ms. A let the therapist know that she and her husband were going to the wedding. The therapist acknowledged that she and her husband would also be there.

After the wedding there was a small reception dinner. The hostess did not know that Ms. A was in treatment with the therapist, and they were seated next to each other at a table for eight. The therapist was in the awkward position of dealing with the conversation at the table and her relationship to Ms. A. During dinner a heated debate occurred, with one of the guests vigorously condemning abortion as "murder." The therapist was aware that Ms. A, who was still dealing with the aftereffects of an abortion, was taking it all in. It was clear that this conversation was going to have adverse effects on Ms. A and would exacerbate her deep feelings of guilt and low self-esteem.

Although the therapist was careful to only listen during this conversation, Ms. A predictably distorted the reality of what occurred. She projected her self-critical perspective and feelings of guilt onto the therapist in the form of an intensified negative transference. At the next session, Ms. A and the therapist reviewed the incident. The strong therapeutic alliance enabled the therapist to assist Ms. A in understanding her distortions, eventually resulting in a resolution of her depression.

In Case 1, the unavoidable social situation was used by the therapist in a professional manner to assist her patient. In contrast, Case 2 illustrates a similar situation in which the therapist and patient attended the same social event, but an unfortunate outcome resulted.

Case 2

A therapist chose not to disclose his intention to attend the same social event his patient, Ms. B, was attending. When the party occurred, Ms. B was surprised to see her therapist present and approached him to engage in social conversation. The therapist attempted to avoid Ms. B and did not acknowledge her greeting, fearing that he might compromise her confidentiality. Subsequently, Ms. B became quite depressed and stopped talking in her therapy hours. The therapist did not understand why she was behaving this way and attributed her behavior to resistance. He had no awareness of his own rejecting behavior at the party. Shortly afterward Ms. B left therapy.

The therapist in Case 2 believed that his avoidance of social contact with Ms. B was a way of maintaining separation between professional and personal roles in the community. He believed that his behavior was consistent with traditional psychodynamic theory and that he was protecting his patient's confidentiality. However, further inquiry revealed that this therapist had strong personal feelings about Ms. B that played a role in the therapy. In not acknowledging their mutual invitation in advance of the event, he had not given Ms. B the opportunity to discuss her fantasies about meeting the therapist or to deal with the extratherapeutic reality. It is likely that the therapist may have acted out his own countertransferential attitudes of rejection and a wish to distance himself from the emotional life of his patient. The effect of the therapist's behavior was to intensify his patient's already considerable self-critical attitudes.

In contrast to the therapist in Case 1, the therapist in Case 2 did not differentiate between a rigid interpretation of proper therapeutic technique and an understanding of his patient's dynamics. Indeed, he used traditional techniques to unconsciously justify his countertransferential feelings about Ms. B. To further compound matters, he did not understand or accept the realities of practicing and living in a small community and therefore would not acknowledge the fact that he and his patients would continue to meet outside of the professional domain.

The small community setting may promote transference distortions during the therapy or even before treatment commences. If the therapist is remarkable in any way, this becomes widely known in both the lay and professional community. The therapist's image in the community may determine whether or not he or she gets referrals or loses patients. This phenomenon may be characterized as a "community transference" or, more accurately, the transference resistance preceding the therapy. Because of the constant crossover of roles within the community, it is common for there to be distortions and idealizations about the therapist long before the therapy starts. This issue also relates to the lack of anonymity we discuss below.

The psychoanalytic literature conveys the impression that perfect therapies are conducted all the time by relying solely on interpretative techniques. It is assumed that personal and professional aspects of one's life should never cross and that all aspects of the transference occur only in the consultation room. Anything less or different is not only unacceptable, but is viewed as if the therapist had compromised himself or herself. This dogmatic perspective is ironic because it is well known that the overlapping of personal and professional roles is an unavoidable aspect of life in a psychoanalytic institute (Kernberg 1986).

The dynamic therapist in a small town is similarly in the difficult position of having to conduct a highly private, confidential dialogue, while, at the same time, both patient and therapist may have frequent extratherapeutic contacts. Practice in a small community is a bit like the story of the emperor who wore no clothes. Everyone knows what is going on, but no one—patient or therapist—feels comfortable acknowledging the mutual exposures.

Confidentiality

The sine qua non of therapy is confidentiality. Without it, the basic foundation of therapy is compromised. All therapists know this, yet there are rare cases in which this may be violated. In a small community it may be very difficult or impossible to maintain the absoluteness of this commitment (Copans and Racusin 1983; Hargrove 1986; Jeffrey and Reeve 1978). Confidentiality may be broken by the patient or the therapist, either accidentally or intentionally.

In a small community there are times when patients talk about their therapy and their therapists. Through a series of conversations the content of these remarks may become distorted. For example, the community gossip may suggest that the therapist is discussing confidential aspects of his patient's treatment when this has never been the case. This can be a serious matter, as is illustrated in the following case example of "community transference":

Case 3

Ms. C, a young patient, came to her therapy hour in an extremely agitated state, saying that she had heard from a colleague that the therapist had divulged that she was in treatment. Furthermore, Ms. C stated that she had been told that the therapist had revealed the time and frequency of appointments. Understandably, she felt that this was a clear violation of confidentiality. Although the therapist had occasional contacts with the colleague, he had never discussed any of his patients. In therapy, the principle of confidentiality was again clarified. The therapist attempted to explore Ms. C's fantasies and community gossip about the therapist, yet Ms. C did not want to explore the matter further.

Therapists may have to address even more delicate matters that occur everyday in a small community. For example, a severely dis-

turbed patient may be a school teacher, nurse, doctor, or other professional who interacts with members of the therapist's family. What is the
proper course that protects everyone's interests in such cases? The therapist is confronted by his or her own multiple allegiances because the
nature of the community does not permit separation of social systems.

Many of the therapists we interviewed reported that sometimes it
was necessary to tell their spouse the name of a patient to bring the
relationship into an appropriate perspective and thereby avoid more
serious violations of confidentiality. Although this intentional and limited breach of confidentiality was felt to be necessary, it was not without risk. The potential benefits of this approach need to be carefully
weighed against the potential harms of violating absolute standards of
confidentiality. For example, in cases where the spouse might not understand the seriousness of maintaining strict name confidentiality, the
consequences of this violation can be destructive for patient and therapist alike. In contrast, the following case example illustrates a limited
breach of confidentiality that successfully averts a harmful event for
the patients while minimizing the risk for further disclosure:

Case 4

A therapist and his family were about to leave for a vacation. It was their
custom to notify the police before they went away. When the therapist's
wife offered to call the police chief, Mr. D, it became necessary for the
therapist to intervene. Mr. D had recently entered therapy and was
suffering from a persistent suspiciousness that severely impaired his
personal and professional judgment. The therapist was concerned that
Mr. D would misinterpret the intent of the call and that this might exacerbate his paranoid fantasies and compromise his therapy. Yet, the therapist had to explain to his wife the reason for his abrupt intervention. The
wife fully understood the delicateness of the matter and that in certain
special situations she was involved in the confidential aspect of her
husband's practice.

Some therapists reported that they discussed issues of confidentiality and conduct in social settings during the first session of treatment
with their patients. This discussion included explicit agreements about
how, or if, their patients would prefer to be greeted in chance meetings
outside of therapy. These therapists appeared more comfortable with a
structure, procedure, and ground rules. In contrast, other therapists,
particularly those who were analytically trained, felt strongly that extratherapeutic contacts should be discussed as they occurred, in the
context of an emerging transference.

Regardless of the therapist's technical approach to the management of confidentiality and transference, it seems essential that an affirmative attitude toward the patient be maintained. If the patient has requested that he or she not be acknowledged in a social setting, this does not permit the therapist to behave in a rude or rejecting manner. On the other hand, acknowledging the patient in a social setting may foster therapy by assisting the patient in recognizing the difference between transferential and real aspects of their relationship. Yet, the open familiarity that is part of living in a small town must be clearly differentiated from any activities that directly threaten the patient's fundamental confidentiality. In small communities it can be assumed that if a therapist divulges any aspect related to a patient's care, both the content and the act itself may quickly become public knowledge.

Anonymity

The therapist who lives and works in the small community cannot be anonymous, as anonymity is contrary to the social structure (Moffic 1981; Riggs and Kugel 1976; Van Dyke 1986). Most therapists, whether living in an urban or small community setting, are involved in activities outside their professional work. In a small community these involvements quickly become known. Based in part on such knowledge, members of the community make judgments about the therapist's personal life-style, values, and interests. As matters of common knowledge, a therapist's social activities, religious practices, politics, and even neighbors may come into the therapy. Therefore, the therapeutic field is rarely neutral and undistorted. Is it possible under these circumstances to practice psychodynamic psychotherapy?

Most of the therapists we interviewed reported that dynamic therapy can be practiced in a small town, but that it requires modification of certain traditional practices, which in turn has theoretical implications. The practice of dynamic therapy in small communities suggests that the transference can occur in a less anonymous field than was previously thought. Whereas the concept of absolute anonymity is appropriate to the urban setting in which social and spatial separations are the norm, a more relativistic concept of anonymity is appropriate to the small community setting. The practice of dynamic therapy in small communities suggests that, to compensate for the absence of spatial and social separation, therapists must rely on their technical skills and emotional control perhaps even more fully than their urban counterparts to achieve therapeutic success. Moreover, therapists in small communities must draw on their own psychological resources to protect themselves from the interference of the therapy with their own private lives. The stress that therapists face personally and professionally be-

cause of the absence of anonymity in small communities is exemplified
by the following case example:

Case 5

Therapist E, who worked in a small community, became seriously ill and
was rushed to the local medical center. Time was critical as she suffered
from a severe hemorrhage related to a gynecological problem. The closest
similarly equipped hospital was 2 hours away.

From the moment Therapist E learned she that was being admitted to
the hospital, she had to think of her behavior and how this would affect
many of her patients who were on the staff or were interns at the medical
center. While in the emergency room she attempted to deal with her fear
of becoming critically ill, while at the same time feeling apprehensive
about being recognized by those who treated her. In all likelihood she
would have to deal with staff members who were her patients.

At one point it looked as if Therapist E might need emergency surgery.
She tried to take her mind off of her anxiety primarily by watching television and reading murder mysteries. There she was, watching "The
Young and the Restless" and wondering if one of her patients would
wander in. She was in the unique position of being a patient in the presence of her own patients.

Finally the day arrived when Therapist E was waiting for her doctor
to come in and tell her the results of the biopsy. Although preliminary
reports suggested that her condition was probably benign, she feared the
worst. Just before her attending physician came in, one of her patients,
who was an intern from another service, stopped in to visit. Although the
conversation was brief, it was long enough for the intern to divulge that
he had read her chart. Therapist E was very upset but had to appear
composed, while trying not to wonder if the intern knew good or bad
news. Further, she had to deal with her feelings of outrage at having her
privacy violated by the intern-patient.

Because there is little separation of social systems in a small community, one can abruptly find oneself in a stressful situation where there
may be a complete role reversal. In Case 5, Therapist E experienced this
crossover as a traumatic event. During her convalescence she was left
to recover both physically and emotionally. In particular, she had to
personally address an intense and potentially destructive countertransference reaction. After personally examining and identifying these responses, she was able to resume treatment and constructively address
the patient's inappropriate violation of her privacy within the therapy.

Unlike the practitioner in an urban setting, the small town therapist
is vulnerable to unanticipated interactions with patients that can result
in countertransference crises. If the therapist cannot accept these possi-

ble realities and understand that transference and countertransference will be experienced "in vivo," he or she may find practicing and living in a small community quite difficult. Another potential liability associated with the lack of anonymity in a small town is illustrated by the following example of a patient with a primitive personality disorder who developed an eroticized transference:

Case 6

Therapist F was treating a borderline patient with hysterical features who developed an intense eroticized transference. In the small town, the patient seemed to pop up everywhere she went, including the supermarket, the one elementary school, the church, and the one major shopping center. Even more private activities were subject to intrusion by her patient. For example, Therapist F regularly went swimming and used the Nautilus machines at a local health club. This had become the highlight of her day and a pleasant escape from the rigors of a busy private practice. The patient eventually joined the club and frequently appeared at her regular exercise time and attempted to engage in conversation. He expressed a wish to know everything about her life and often inquired about her spouse and her children.

Therapist F addressed her patient's transference and behavior in therapy, but she was unable to intervene successfully. He insisted that he was "in love" with her and refused to alter his attempts to see her outside the therapeutic hour. Setting limits on his violation of her privacy was complicated by the lack of options in the small town setting. Her patient insisted that many of the meetings were coincidental and reflected the realities of life in a small town. Therapist F and her family felt like they were being besieged. The whole town knew by this time that the patient was in treatment with her. After considerable effort and unsuccessful attempts to work through the eroticized transference, she transferred the patient to another therapist leaving him enraged and just as determined.

After several months of continuing to run into the patient around town, Therapist F decided to move to another town to get away from this stress. Whereas she used to be able to walk to her office (and her husband could walk or bike to his), they both now had to drive to their offices 45 minutes away, and their children had to transfer to another school.

We are all familiar with the demands of practice, especially of treating patients with primitive character disorders. In Case 6, we are confronted with a situation in which the reality of the small community seemed to exacerbate acting-out in primitive personalities. This set of circumstances could easily lead to a disastrous set of therapeutic circumstances. In our discussions with therapists, there was a general consensus that dynamically oriented psychotherapy of primitive personality disorders presented special risks in the small community. As patients with primitive personality disorders characteristically distort the differentiation between the real and the transferential relationship, the treatment of such patients in a setting where there is already an inadequate spatial and social separation between a therapist's personal and professional life can become an enormous challenge. The psychological compensation that therapists in the small community setting must provide themselves when treating all patients may not be enough when an intense and eroticized transference develops in a seriously disturbed patient.

Adjustment to Practice in a Small Town

Making the move.   What would lead a dynamic therapist to move to a small community? Our discussions with therapists suggest that most decided to move for personal reasons with little prior appreciation for the realities of small town practice. The difficulties of adjusting to this move may dramatically surface when private and professional responsibilities collide. This conflict is demonstrated in the following example:

Case 7

Therapist G, a 35-year-old psychologist, was trained at a large, urban clinical psychology program, well known for its focus on dynamically oriented psychotherapy. After practicing for several years in an urban group practice, she moved with her husband and her young son to a small New England town where she joined a community clinic practice. Both she and her husband had discussed this move for some time and had fantasized about bringing up their child in a safe, contained environment.

One of Therapist G's first patients was a female school teacher who entered into weekly psychotherapy for anxiety and low self-esteem. Much of the treatment focused on addressing her anger toward her mother, whom she experienced as unavailable and incompetent. In the course of the therapy, a maternal transference developed with Therapist G, which allowed for a favorable therapeutic context to work through these events.

Therapist G had some personal difficulty in adjusting to her move to a small town, and she particularly felt that her son had also experienced difficulty in making the transition. In planning for her son's schooling for the next year, Therapist G realized that her patient was to be her son's teacher. This teacher was well known as the best of the teachers at the son's grade level. The anticipation of discussing her son's performance and adjustment problems with her patient in parent conferences presented a complex dilemma that could directly affect the work of the therapy. Conversely, asking for a reassignment to a different teacher would be awkward and would threaten the patient's confidentiality. Furthermore, Therapist G's son would be deprived of the best educational opportunity.

Eventually, Therapist G decided to transfer her patient to another therapist and to keep her son in the assigned class. Discussion of this decision in the therapy was limited, reflecting Therapist G's discomfort with the situation. Ultimately, she felt that her own priorities as a mother had displaced the needs of her patient. The therapy ended with both patient and therapist experiencing many unresolved feelings. Their future relationship as mother and teacher was awkward and distant.

It seems that younger, less experienced therapists, trained in urban programs, are inadequately prepared for the change in the therapeutic paradigm that they have so recently learned. Perhaps their recently established identities as therapists have not yet been sufficiently integrated and personalized through experience to permit yet another adjustment. They tend to be inflexible and to feel exposed. The difficulties with adjustment are generally denied, and the differences from the urban environment are not acknowledged. The following case example illustrates a contrasting experience, described by a senior therapist who decided to move from the suburbs of a large city to the country:

Case 8

Therapist H had a large psychoanalytic practice in a New York suburban area. He looked forward to more regular hours and not being subject to commuter schedules in order to maintain his practice. He moved to a small town in Vermont where he enjoyed seeing his patients around town and in different settings and perspectives. He took comfort in this greater sense of continuity with his community. He was overwhelmed at first by the crossover of social roles and the frequent contact patients would have with his wife. This had never occurred in his former practice in New York.

However, Therapist H was quite resourceful and was able to recognize that, although this was stressful, he had an opportunity to reassess his ideas about what helped in therapy. He realized that such inadvertent contacts did not lead to negative therapeutic results as he had been taught in practice. Gradually and painfully, he went through a transformation and developed a new view of his role as a therapist. He became less confined by theory and more open to new ideas. Interestingly, he realized that his previous environment had unknowingly affected his clinical thinking.

For some therapists a small community may foster fantasies of an extended family and a concept of safety. Perhaps for some therapists the small community can be viewed as a form of selfobject transference that supports both the therapists and their patients. These therapists may be more comfortable with a two-party therapeutic paradigm in which the transference is viewed in the here and now (Loewald 1960). Favorable adjustments to practice in a small community clearly reflect a combination of factors, including therapists' personality, theoretical orientation, and clinical experience.

With the exception of those who trained locally, we found that most therapists decided to move from urban settings to small communities for personal reasons. They were largely unaware of the potential impact of the small community on themselves, their therapeutic techniques, and paradigms of therapeutic effectiveness. These therapists felt unprepared for the realities of small town practice and found that the impact of setting and community on their personal and professional lives was enormous.

Social isolation. Isolation is a factor that confronts almost all psychotherapists because the work is by nature quite solitary. This is true in both the urban setting and the small community. It would be extremely difficult for a therapist living in a small community to maintain total anonymity and have any kind of personal or professional life. Indeed, this is especially true for unmarried therapists and for younger therapists who have recently moved from an urban area (Riggs and Kugel 1976). The former are isolated by virtue of their marital status and have fewer opportunities to meet appropriate mates. The need for isolation and the impact of that isolation can be devastating to the therapist. The following case examples highlight this issue:

Case 9

Therapist J, a single woman, moved from New York City to Vermont because of an unusual professional opportunity. However, she did not fully realize that it would be difficult to establish an active social life. In New York she could socialize widely with professional impunity. However, in her new, small community she was shocked to meet many of her single patients at the local dance spots. She recognized that she could not mix her personal and professional lives. She was forced to commute to New York on weekends. Therapist J realized that without a social life, she would not be able to function professionally. Most of her professional colleagues were married, and although friendly, did not invite her to dinner parties. After several years of depression, she moved back to New York.

The unusual position of being a therapist in a small town can affect the way that one is perceived as a member of the social community. The reaction of friends and acquaintances is described in the following case example:

Case 10

Therapist K, a 32-year-old woman who had worked for 6 years as a therapist, "retired" to be at home full time with her children. Seven years later, when her youngest child entered first grade, she decided to resume her clinical practice in her hometown. During her "retirement," she had a full social life in the community. She was very visible. Interestingly, her friends were surprised to learn that she had been a therapist before having children.

As Therapist K's practice and identity as a therapist solidified, she observed that she experienced subtle changes in her personal relationships. For example, a number of her friends wanted her to offer therapeutic help. Furthermore, she learned from her patients and professional colleagues confidential information about these friends that she had not previously known. Therapist K became increasingly uncomfortable and realized that she had to be more discriminating in her friendships. By her second year of practice, her circle of friends had largely changed to professional colleagues.

Some of the therapists who had recently moved from urban areas reported a need for greater structuring of treatment than they had previously experienced. This bolstering of the separation between real and transferential aspects of the therapy by reinforcing the "rules" of good therapy has personal consequences for therapists. Actively avoiding all situations where extratherapeutic contacts with patients might occur restricts participation in the community and adds to discomfort in circumstances involving one's children, medical care, religious, and community functions. It can be done, but at a price that would not be as exacting in an urban setting. Importantly, older, more experienced therapists seem to be less concerned about this. As one senior therapist said, "As I got older and more senior, I felt more confident about my role in the community and felt less concerned about the need to be isolated or protected from extratherapeutic contacts." These factors of isolation and the need for personal privacy may be critical whether or not a therapist remains in the community. Indeed they could play a role in the shaping of the therapist's professional interests away from clinical work.

The problems that social isolation may present can be serious for the therapist who feels that contact of any type with patients outside of therapy represents a "contaminant." If this therapist does not enjoy rural isolation and cannot collect a coterie of similarly minded colleagues, personal and professional survival may be impossible. On the other hand, most therapists interviewed seemed to integrate their personal and professional lives by using the psychological defenses of isolation and adaptive denial. The ability to divorce and repress one's affect may play an important role in appropriately and objectively adapting to the reality of practice in a small community.

A strict ideologue who believes that therapeutic technique will assure absolute technical neutrality and anonymity may underestimate how the urban environment protects and facilitates this model of treatment. The urban setting provides complete isolation for the practice of dynamic therapy without imposing a similar social isolation that would make such work virtually impossible. The therapist living and practicing in the small town cannot isolate practice from life in the community. We found that many therapists felt somewhat restricted in their social activities and relationships. Many relied heavily on family or a small network of friends. The therapist who lacks a protected network of fulfilling relationships is particularly vulnerable to severe isolation and demoralization.

REASSESSING BASIC PRINCIPLES AND ASSUMPTIONS OF DYNAMIC PSYCHOTHERAPY

The dynamic therapist who lives and works in a small community is faced with a unique set of problems. The small town therapist is not protected by the customary mantle of anonymity, isolation, and the separation of professional and personal roles. Instead, the therapist is thrown entirely on psychological resources to maintain the therapeutic environment with little support from the surroundings. These factors require that the therapist modify technical aspects of therapeutic style without sacrificing ideals and ethical standards of properly conducted therapy.

The overlapping of social systems in a small community expose therapists to frequent opportunities for countertransference distortions and acting out. The need to be aware of this is essential. The blurring of boundaries and roles that is part of small town practice requires that therapists particularly be aware of the potential for unethical and destructive behavior. Frequent consultation and peer supervision (if available) are vital resources for addressing problematic situations as they occur. In addition, the therapist must be especially sensitive to personal and professional vulnerabilities associated with countertransference. The therapist without adequate psychodynamic therapy may be at increased risk in a small community.

Moreover, the persistence of overlapping social systems has a tendency to force the therapist to use therapeutic paradigms that involve the therapist more actively. This therapy may be more of an open two-party system with a focus on aspects of the transference experience in the here and now. This may include dealing with material directly relating to the therapist's life in the community. The therapist who is willing to practice in a small community may be unconscious of these factors, yet personally may be more comfortable with a flexible approach to treatment and the absence of clear boundaries. On the other hand, there are therapists in the community who feel the need to be quite structured and formal in their therapeutic techniques to minimize the impact of the small community on their professional work. They, too, may be unaware of the full impact of the small community on their therapeutic technique.

Several preliminary observations have emerged from our interviews with small town therapists. Some degree of flexibility in conducting therapy appears to be essential to surviving as a therapist in a small community. Extratherapeutic contact with patients is inevitable and therefore must be integrated into the experience of therapy. Although the therapist cannot be a neutral mirror for the elaboration of the transference, he or she can maintain a neutral therapeutic attitude. As some have suggested, the relationship between the patient and the therapist may be the most essential component of treatment, and specific techniques such as interpretation of the transference may be less important (Luborsky 1984). There may be, in fact, more opportunity for appropriate flexibility without sacrificing the best traditions of good dynamic therapy.

It may be argued that if traditional techniques and practices of dynamic psychotherapy were absolutely essential, it would be impossible to treat patients in a small community. From our interviews of therapists, we found no evidence to suggest that the quality and outcome of therapy was significantly affected by compromises resulting from the small town setting. Perhaps some of the traditional principles of dynamic therapy are not as vital as previously held. For example, anonymity of the therapist, the elaboration of an uncontaminated transference, and the absence of crossover of social and professional roles may be epiphenomena. In fact, it is even possible that they may hamper the therapy and prolong unresolved transferences. Perhaps an appropriate emphasis on the therapeutic alliance as reinforced by the community actually fosters the therapeutic process.

It should be emphasized that none of the therapists interviewed felt that adopting a flexible therapeutic stance justified any compromise in basic standards of ethical behavior. For example, flexibility should not be confused with befriending, employing, or having a sexual involvement with a patient. These activities are unethical and have destructive effects on the patient and the therapist. Allowing for extratherapeutic contacts and flexibility in technique is, instead, a recognition of the reality of conducting psychotherapy in a small town setting.

Historically, it was necessary for therapists to believe that their paradigmatic model of mental illness was correct and absolute, and therefore the technique, if followed, would lead to the etiological basis of the disorder. In this context, the rigid adherence to technique was justified. Another possibility worthy of consideration is that rigid adherence to technique was used in a countertransferential dimension by the therapist, in order not to interact appropriately with the patient. Thus the application of the theoretical technique became more important than the patient, sometimes at the expense of the therapy.

The idea that the structural theory is the only correct psychoanalytic model is no longer held. It is clear that all dynamic therapists, knowingly or otherwise, use a series of models and techniques. There has been a gradual shift to a utilization of a variety of techniques that include, but are not limited to, interpretation. The psychodynamic literature now acknowledges the possibility for multiple etiologies of neurotic disorders, including biological contributions. Psychodynamic therapy therefore is more flexible and accurate without sacrificing ideals. Issues of technique are no longer seen as synonymous with models of mental disorder or their etiology. Indeed, a broader view of emotional disorders within psychodynamic therapy has led to a variety of techniques (Simons 1990).

The natural overlapping of social systems within the small community and the consequent demands to be therapeutically flexible are compatible with the movement away from the "myth of perfectibility" (Blum 1989; Gaskill 1980), which for so long has hung over the techniques of psychodynamic therapy. The small community forces us in our daily work to question our idealizations and look more carefully at our ideals. The transference not only develops within the therapy, but is inevitably affected by the reality of small community life. As dynamic therapy has evolved, we now realize and acknowledge that the therapy is, of necessity, a two-party system. No longer is the therapist's stance outside, looking on the action or remaining the inactive sounding board (Loewald 1960). Perhaps, for heuristic purposes, the small community can provide us with a rich opportunity to further our study of how therapists really practice dynamic therapy and which therapeutic factors contribute to more rapid and more effective results.

The therapist who comes to live and practice in a small community must be willing to consider these issues to survive personally and professionally. Recently there has been a striking increase in reference (see Kluft 1989; Simons 1990) to Charcot's famous quote, "Theory is good, but it doesn't prevent things from existing" (see Freud 1893, p. 13). Now, as the whole field of dynamic psychotherapy is opening up to scientific study and the adherence to a solitary paradigm of etiology and technique is dissolving, this observation seems especially appropriate. It is a warning to each of us that we not be blinded by our theories. As Lawrence Friedman (1988) pointed out, our theories may represent the therapist's wishes—the wish to understand, the wish for certainty, and the wish for closure. Our preliminary survey of therapists reemphasizes the need to maintain the priority of clinical observation over theory.

As we mature and try to understand ourselves and our therapeutic behavior, we should not in any way confuse this with the basic contract with our patients, namely, to be their therapist whom they can trust, to not compromise our fundamental ethical standards, and above all "to keep hope alive" (Rodman 1986). These issues remain inviolate regardless of our paradigms. Practice in a small community forces us to acknowledge and do what we have to, within the principles of dynamic psychotherapy. As Elvin Semrad once said, "A therapist is a kind of service man. There are so many things a patient can want to use you for—and if you can swallow your own ideas of how things should be, you can perform a real service" (Rako and Mazer 1980, p. 102).

REFERENCES

Blum HP: The concept of termination and the evolution of psychoanalytic thought. J Am Psychoanal Assoc 37:275–295, 1989

Copans S, Racusin R: Rural child psychiatry. J Am Acad Child Psychiatry 22:184–190, 1983

Freud S: Charcot (1893), in The Standard Edition of the Complete Psychological Works of Sigmund Freud, Vol 3. Edited and translated by Strachey J. London, Hogarth Press, 1962, pp 9–23

Friedman L: The Anatomy of Psychotherapy. Hillsdale, NJ, Analytic Press, 1988

Gaskill HS: The closing phase of the psychoanalytic treatment of adults and the goals of psychoanalysis: "the myth of perfectibility." Int J Psychoanal 61:11–23, 1980

Greenson RR: The working alliance and the transference neurosis. Psychoanal Q 34:155–181, 1965

Greenson RR, Wexler M: The non-transference relationship in the psychoanalytic situation. Int J Psychoanal 50:27–39, 1969

Hargrove DS: An overview of professional considerations in the rural community, in Handbook of Rural Community Mental Health. Edited by Keller PA, Murray JD. New York, Human Sciences Press, 1982, pp 169–182

Hargrove DS: A commentary on rural mental health training, in Innovations in Rural Community Mental Health. Edited by Murray JD, Keller PA. Mansfield, PA, Mansfield University Rural Services Institute, 1986, pp 239–249

Jeffrey MF, Reeve RE: Community mental health in rural areas: some practical issues. Community Ment Health J 14:54–62, 1978

Kernberg O: Institutional problems of psychoanalytic education. J Am Psychoanal Assoc 34:799–834, 1986

Kluft R: Rigid adherence to a theoretical paradigm can hinder therapy. Clinical Psychiatry News 17(5):26, 1989

Loewald H: On the therapeutic action of psychoanalysis. Int J Psychoanal 41:16–33, 1960

Luborsky L: Principles of Psychoanalytic Psychotherapy: A Manual for Supportive-Expressive Treatment. New York, Basic Books, 1984

Mazer M: People and Predicaments. Cambridge, MA, Harvard University Press, 1976

Moffic SH: Therapist anonymity in rural areas. Am J Psychoanal 41:85–89, 1981

Rako S, Mazer H: Semrad: The Heart of a Therapist. New York, Jason Aronson, 1980

Riggs RT, Kugel LF: Transition from urban to rural mental health practice. Social Casework 57:562–567, 1976

Rodman RF: Keeping Hope Alive: On Becoming a Psychotherapist. New York, Harper & Row, 1986

Simons RC: Our analytic heritage: ideals and idealizations. J Am Psychoanal Assoc 38:5–38, 1990

Sterba R: The fate of the ego in analytic therapy. Int J Psychoanal 15:117–126, 1934

Van Dyke DA: The psychiatrist in a rural community, in Innovations in Rural Community Mental Health. Edited by Murray JD, Keller PA. Mansfield, PA, Mansfield University Rural Services Institute, 1986, pp 27–36

Chapter 2

The Vulnerable Therapist:
On Being Ill or Injured

Henry Grunebaum, M.D.

The heartache and the thousand natural shocks that flesh is heir to.

William Shakespeare, *Hamlet*

Having a serious illness or injury is at best a trying ordeal and at worst a tragedy. It is a uniquely personal experience that impinges on those with whom the injured person is most intimately involved, usually family and friends. But when the injured person is a therapist, an illness or injury is also an event shared with his or her patients. In fact, we could not understand our patient's pain and suffering were we not ourselves similarly vulnerable. As the classicist and philosopher Martha Nussbaum has written, "Part of the peculiar beauty of human excellence just is its vulnerability" (Nussbaum 1986, p. 2).

To write this chapter, I reviewed the literature and carried out a small-sample interview study of therapists, asking them about their experiences with illness and injury. What was most memorable in both the literature and the interview accounts was the courage and fortitude of these therapists and their dedication to their patient's well-being. What influence their actions and attitudes had on their patients is perhaps the most important question we can ask if we are to learn how to face such inevitable experiences in life.

However, the questions usually asked when a therapist is ill or injured are "Should one tell one's patients the truth?" and/or "What does one tell one's patients?" In this chapter, I take the position (based on the

I wish to acknowledge the contributions of Judith Grunebaum and Bennett Simon for their careful reading and comments on this chapter. I am also deeply grateful to the 12 therapists who discussed their illnesses with me.

literature and the interview study) that it is best to tell our patients the relevant truth; indeed, there are many good reasons for telling the truth. Moreover, it seems likely that how we think about discussing an illness or injury with patients has general implications about what we should share with patients. I also discuss the far more common predicament that arises when therapists who are physically impaired see their patients. There is, however, one striking lacuna in the literature on therapists' illnesses; there are no case reports by therapists who experienced a psychiatric illness. Obviously, considering estimates that about 10% of men and 20% of women experience a significant depression or manic-depressive illness during their lives (Weissman et al. 1989), psychiatric illness among therapists cannot be uncommon. Indeed, according to Deutsch (1985), 57% of all therapists have been depressed at some time in their lives.

LITERATURE AND INTERVIEWS

Because a literature search revealed only a few case reports, each by a therapist writing about his or her illness and describing its impact on a few patients, and because none of the reports involved more than one therapist (making comparisons difficult), I conducted an interview study of 12 therapists who had dealt with an illness or injury in their own lives. The 12 therapists were found through my personal network of contacts, including names volunteered by colleagues and by the subjects themselves. I called each therapist explaining that I had been asked to write this chapter and that a mutual acquaintance had informed me of his or her illness. I then asked if he or she would be willing to participate in a brief interview. In addition, I told them that they would have an opportunity to read and comment on this chapter, to make sure that it represented their experiences accurately and did not violate their confidentiality. One of the study subjects, Amy L. Morrison, specifically asked me to include her name in the following discussion; her request has been complied with.

The interviews were an effort to learn how the therapists had dealt with illness or injury as it affected their professional lives and were usually conducted in the therapists' homes. I was particularly interested in what they had told their patients, why they had decided to follow a particular course of action, and what the outcome was. Naturally, along the way I learned a good deal about how this event affected their personal lives as well. The nature of the interviews was such that no empathic interviewer would not have been moved by their stories of adversity and courage, and most of the subjects were quite interested in sharing their experiences. In particular, I want to express my gratitude to Amy L. Morrison, a Cambridge psychiatric social worker, who shared a prepublication copy of a chapter she had written (Morrison 1990). It gives a far fuller account than can be given here of the reactions of individual patients to her cancer, how she dealt in therapy with these issues, and her own feelings and reactions to the illness and her patients.

The interview sample included seven psychiatrists (four of whom were also psychoanalysts), two psychologists, and three social workers (Table 2–1). They ranged in age from the early thirties to the early seventies. Several other therapists, all psychoanalysts, declined to be interviewed. Because two of those who declined indicated that they believed their patients did not know about a major illness or a major operation, their absence may skew the findings. Other therapists contacted simply stated that they were too busy or that it would be upsetting to discuss such private matters.

Table 2–1. Characteristics of 12 therapists who sustained illness or injury

Therapist	Sex	Profession	Age	Illness or injury	Visible sequelae
A	M	MD	70+	Cardiac bypass	Weight loss
B	M	Psy	60+	Myocardial infarct	None
C	F	SW	50+	Ovarian cancer	Effects of chemotherapy
D	M	MD	60+	Foot infection	None (saw patients in hospital)
E	F	Psy	40+	Breast cancer	Effects of chemotherapy
F	M	MD*	50+	Severe injury to leg	Limp and cast
G	M	MD*	50+	Hearing loss	Hearing aid
H	M	MD*	60+	Cardiac bypass	None
I	F	MD	30	Wrist surgery	Cast on forearm
J	F	SW	40+	Depression	None (although some patients noticed)
K	M	MD*	50+	Diabetes	None
A. L. M.	F	SW	50+	Breast cancer	Effects of chemotherapy

Note. MD = psychiatrist; MD* = psychiatrist-psychoanalyst;
Psy = psychologist; SW = social worker.

PERSONAL EXPERIENCES

I was not asked to write this chapter as a neutral and disinterested professional, but precisely because I had published a paper describing an experience with an injury many years ago (Grunebaum 1973). At that time, based on a misunderstanding of what a colleague had told me, I decided to see three patients in my hospital room while recovering from a fractured pelvis. I later resumed therapy with most of my private patients in an office in my house and still later in my hospital office while on crutches. During some of this period I was in mild to moderate pain.

Much more recently, I have fractured my right arm twice. The first, a fracture of the radius, was casted and I used a sling. However, 1 week later it required a scheduled operation to provide an external fixator (a device involving four pins screwed into the bones of the forearm and attached to each other by slender metal rods). This apparatus, which looks like something made from an Erector set, was quite visible, although relatively painless. The other fracture, of the head of the humerus, required the use of a sling and was rather painful for a considerable period although the worst of the pain was controlled by aspirin. Other than these injuries, I had only the usual quota of minor illnesses until the summer of 1989 when I had a small basal cell cancer removed from beside my nose.

Clearly, these experiences have influenced my thinking about how to deal with illness or injury in my work. First, except for the surgery, these events were unplanned and unpredictable, and thus it was impossible to prepare my patients in advance. Second, in each instance I was able to resume work while still recovering. Finally, each of the events led to visible consequences.

PARAMETERS OF THE ILLNESS OR INJURY

In any discussion of a therapist's illness or injury, there are several questions about the event that must be considered. I discuss each of these questions below in conjunction with both the interviews and the literature.

Does the Therapist Have Any Notice About What Is to Occur?

A breast biopsy or an coronary bypass can be scheduled, but this is not true for most serious illnesses or injuries, which strike without warning. Thus often it is not possible for us to prepare our patients in advance for an absence. Even scheduled absences can change without warning. For example, Therapist A (a Boston psychiatrist) told his patients of his impending bypass operation. However, he could not tell them about the near fatal complications after the surgery that necessitated a far longer hospital stay than he had planned for and told his patients to expect. His family had to arrange to leave reports on his answering machine to let his patients know what was going on. Clearly, patients will have different reactions to absences that are sudden than they will to ones that are expected.

Who Informs the Patients?

Some of the therapists informed their patients of their injuries and illnesses themselves. For example, Abend (1982), a psychoanalyst, wrote, "There was a substantial interval between the establishment of the diagnosis and the actual institution of treatment, during which I was able to continue working, so there was ample opportunity for me to consult with colleagues about how best to handle the situation" (p. 365). Likewise, in my case, even though the accident occurred (by very nature) without warning, I was initially able to explain to my patients in person that the cast I was wearing was for a fracture that had occurred over the previous weekend. Later I could prepare them for the scheduled surgery.

Sometimes the therapist is able to decide what others will say. For example, Dewald (1982), a psychoanalyst, was well enough to tell his secretary to tell his patients at first that he was "ill in the hospital," then that he "was still in the hospital but hoped to be back at work the following week," and finally that he "would be away from [his] practice indefinitely and would contact them when . . . ready to return" (p. 349). Another example is that of Therapist B (a Boston psychologist), who had a mild myocardial infarct and discussed with his wife how she should tell his patients the facts of his illness.

Not every therapist who experiences an illness or injury, however, is fortunate enough to be able to tell their patients themselves or decide what is to be said by others. Often in the midst of an emergency, spouses and/or secretaries have to decipher illegible entries in appointment books in order to inform patients, and some patients may come to an appointment, only to find a note on the office door or the office door simply locked. As Dewald (1982) wrote, "At the height of my illness, decisions were made and communicated to the patients by people other than myself, who would not be in a position to know or anticipate the transference reactions" (p. 350).

How Long Will It Take to Recover?

Brief episodes are relatively easy to deal with but longer absences may require different approaches. It may be necessary to provide alternative coverage if one is going to be out for a prolonged period. On the other hand, the unpredictability of the course of illness and injury must be acknowledged. Patients react differently to short absences, which are commonplace (e.g., an absence due to the flu), than they do to long interruptions of treatment. Indeed, an absence due to a vacation may well be considerably longer than one due to a serious illness; the difference is that in illness or injury the therapist is perceived to be vulnerable rather than enjoying life. Patients do not react simply to the absence of their therapist, they also react to the reason for the absence.

How Serious Is the Illness or Injury?

An illness or injury with an uncertain or fatal prognosis is particularly difficult to confront. In such situations, the therapist and his or her friends and family, colleagues, and patients will have to deal with issues of how they confront not simply absence, but death. Facing death is quite different from facing a case with less threatening illnesses or injuries. However, in either event, the patient must deal with the vulnerabilities of the therapist.

Meloche (1984), a social worker, described the case of her good friend and colleague Jean Caron, a 39-year-old psychiatrist, who developed and died of leukemia. It took Meloche, "nearly five years of mourning and inner elaboration to be able to organize this experience in its definitive form" (p. 332). She wrote a very moving account of Caron's terminal leukemia and how he dealt with his patients with honesty and courage (Meloche 1984).

Therapists do not want to make patients needlessly anxious, but the anger and sense of betrayal of patients who felt deceived in believing that things were not serious when they were has been described by therapists citing both personal experience and reports of patients. For example, a patient was told by her analyst that she was terminating her practice to "have more time for herself," but the patient learned from her new therapist that the analyst had actually been dying and later had died. The patient felt "horribly betrayed" and it took years for her to regain trust in therapists.

How different was the experience of Jean Caron's patients (Meloche 1984). Some of them found out accidentally that he was terminally ill; others he told himself. He said to one, "But you know I am sick. If I were sick and didn't tell you about it, you would feel cheated once more, as you have always been" (p. 334). And, "You can talk to me who will die shortly, as you could not talk to your mother who is already dead" (p. 334). The effect of this on many of his patients was remarkable. One of Caron's patient who had always run away from emotionally charged situations got involved in the care of his dying brother and told Caron, "To allow others to be present at one's death is to make them a priceless present" (p. 333).

How Predictable Is the Outcome?

Some illnesses and injuries usually result in total recovery, but others often involve a prolonged recovery and prolonged treatment. Still others often lead to some permanent impairment that does not interfere with the ability to work but does influence it. Finally, others are fatal.

I will not spend much time discussing the fact that therapists, like everyone else, should, but do not, make detailed preparations for what should be done were they to become suddenly ill or die. As Guy and Souder (1986) noted, "Taking steps to anticipate or prepare for the impact of eventual illness, injury, or death on one's therapy practice feels much like purchasing family burial plots in advance" (p. 512). Nonetheless, most therapists, like other people, write wills and take appropriate action to protect their families. Although making such preparations with regard to one's patients seems like a good idea, not having taken these steps myself, I cannot in good conscience urge other to do so. Perhaps most therapists are engaging in a denial of the effects of their death on their patients, who are surely vulnerable. However, perhaps none of us can face the "whole truth"; there may be limits to what can be faced while living a livable life.

Much of what is written assumes that the outcome of an illness can be predicted. Often both the duration and outcome are totally unpredictable. A good example of this was provided by Dewald (1982), who thought he had a mild virus. His illness, however, turned out to be meningoencephalitis resulting in a cavernous sinus thrombosis and necessitating a lengthy hospitalization. Because of nerve damage, he returned to work wearing a patch over his eye. The case of Therapist A (who had complications from cardiac bypass surgery) also illustrates the unpredictability of illness and its treatment.

What Are the Sequelae of the Illness or Injury and How Apparent Are They?

It may or may not be apparent to the patient when a therapist is injured or ill. However, a fractured arm in a sling, a hearing aid, special

glasses, or marked loss of weight are visible, and the therapist is likely
to be asked what happened. Sometimes therapists will "give themselves away" simply by the manner of their comments. Morrison
(1990) found herself seeing a patient who "also was awaiting the results of a breast biopsy. She detected from the knowingness of my comments and I allowed, that I was in the 'same boat' . . . and I experienced
the coincidence as both serendipitous and bonding" (p. 232). The patient also experienced "a sense of closeness," but ultimately, because of
differences in the course of their conditions, the patient had to "discon-
nect" from the therapy.

   On the other hand, only some of Morrison's patients seemed to notice that she was wearing a wig during a course of chemotherapy, and
Therapist C (a psychiatric social worker and couples therapist), who
was also on chemotherapy, had a patient comment to her, "I love your
new hairdo." Caron had a similar experience; as Meloche (1984) wrote,
"Thus when Caron's hair went quickly from flaming red to pale ash
blond, nobody mentioned it" (p. 333). However, all of Hannett's patients guessed accurately that her sudden 2-week absence was due to a
miscarriage (Hannett 1949). How many patients have noticed changes
in their therapist but not commented for conscious or unconscious reasons is, of course, unknown.

When Do Patients Learn About the Illness, What Do They Learn, and What Is Their Reaction?

Almost all therapists, to judge from the literature and the interviews,
tell their patients something about their illness or injury unless they
are too ill. Dewald (1982) noted the advantages of being able to decide
what to tell and thus to know what was said. On the other hand, some
of Caron's patients learned about his terminal illness from a television
interview he gave, even though he was disguised, because his voice
was not changed. These patients were quite troubled, unlike those he
had already told himself. He explained to the patients why he had appeared on television and apologized for not being able to inform them
in advance (Meloche 1984).

   Patients have a variety of reactions to such news. Some have the
usual and expectable reactions to a particular illness, whereas others
have reactions that are quite idiosyncratic and based on their own lives.
Three of my patients had sessions with me while I was hospitalized
with a fractured pelvis (Grunebaum 1973). One patient, a middle-aged
mental health professional commented on arriving that she should
have brought me something but hardly mentioned my injury. The hour
seemed little different from previous sessions. In the following hour,

however, she brought a bottle of sherry and related a dream during which she had wept. She knew the dream had to do with my illness and in particular her feeling that there was really nothing that I had expected from her in the hour. I had made no demands, and indeed there was nothing she needed to do or could have done for me because I was well cared for. She felt that this was one of the first times in her life in which she had not felt burdened by a close human relationship and went on to relate how she had been able to offer assistance spontaneously to one of her children without asking for anything in return, a very new experience for her.

Another patient, a young school teacher, appeared with two gifts: a chrysanthemum, "for your soul," and a chocolate sundae, "for your body." We then discussed quite briefly the facts of my injury, much as one would with a friend. There was a pause, and I asked her how she was. She referred to the fact that in a session 1 month before, I had commented that sometimes one had the right to be angry at someone even when something had happened that could not have been helped. She realized now that she was angry with me and that it was all right to be angry.

The third patient, a 24-year-old hospital worker from a housing project who had a very deprived childhood, brought me two Oreo cookies from an opened package. She discussed her inability to express her positive feelings and was quite aware of her anger at me. She wondered if I would find her burdensome and felt I had no positive feelings about her. We discussed her difficulties in expressing positive feelings, and she confided that earlier in the hour she had wished to come over, put her hand on my shoulder, and wish me well. At that point she was able to come over and take my hand and say goodbye. She subsequently sent me a get-well card and began to express positive feelings in other relationships.

Each of the patient's gifts could be understood in terms of the dynamics of that patient and were discussed as it seemed appropriate. After my discharge from the hospital about 1 month later, all three patients reported that they had found seeing me in the hospital useful. They experienced me as "more human," which made it easier to talk to me. In addition (as discussed at greater length below), exploring in therapy how each of these patients felt about being concerned about me and my pain turned out to be invaluable. It gave both of us a chance to see a different side of the patient.

Dewald (1982) had a different experience when his patients, having been informed of his illness and where he was hospitalized, "sent cards, flowers, or other signs of interest, concern, and sympathy . . . some offered advice about treatment . . . [and] some came to his room"

(p. 350). The severity of his illness created a problem because his wife had to acknowledge the cards and gifts. He noted that "since she had not personally experienced the therapeutic process and the nature and meanings of transference reactions, the feelings expressed in these ways by the patients became a source of some conflict and misunderstanding for her, thus indirectly increasing the countertransference implications for me. . . . But to remain abstinent and not acknowledge the patient's gestures would also have affected the therapeutic process" (p. 350–351).

Dewald's report (1982) is unusual in that he described the actions and feelings of his wife and their implications for him. On the other hand, the wife of the Therapist A was his cotherapist and thus involved with many of his patients. She undertook the responsibility for putting messages on his answering machine about his progress. The literature provides no other descriptions of what the therapist's spouse and family do during the illness or injury in relation to his or her practice. Yet this must be quite common (i.e., spouses must often assume unexpected responsibilities for ill or injured therapists). Probably therapists feel more comfortable about describing their own experiences than those of their loved ones.

Oesterheld and Buckman (1989) offered a useful typology of the aspects of a therapist's illnesses or injuries that "trigger transference reactions." These aspects include 1) the absence of the therapist due to illness or injury, 2) the perceived vulnerability of the therapist, 3) the manifestations of the therapist's medical illness or injury, and 4) particular symptoms of the therapist's illness or injury that evoke idiosyncratic reactions. The authors gave examples of patient transference reactions to each of these aspects of illness or injury in the therapist. The scheme I propose in this chapter emphasizes some other aspects of the illness or injury, but Oesterheld and Buckman's typology is valuable in its clarity and simplicity.

THERAPIST VARIABLES

Desire and Need of the Therapist to Work

The literature and interviews were in striking agreement on the subject of therapists' desire and need to return to work. All therapists want to go back to work, not surprisingly, because doing psychotherapy or psychoanalysis is a vital and enjoyable part of their identity. Other motives therapists have for working include self-esteem, the need to prove oneself competent and intact, fears and anxieties, and (as with other self-employed individuals) the fact that income depends directly on the number of hours worked. Givelber and Simon (1981) discussed the grieving therapist's needs for closeness and intimacy and the desire for "business as usual," feelings that are also true for the convalescing therapist. Finally, therapists respond to their guilt about neglecting patients' needs. As Dewald (1982) noted, "The genuine needs of the patients, some of which were communicated by letter or telephone, served to encourage resumption of practice" (p. 352).

Therapists seem to need to get back to work, perhaps even a little too soon, as I did. At the time, I wrote that "the other side of my conflict was equally distressing. Perhaps I was acting in a foolhardy fashion, extending my limits inappropriately in order to test them and myself" (Grunebaum 1973, p. 41). Givelber and Simon (1981) noted that a therapist who has experienced a familial death, a not dissimilar situation, often feels that "he or she should be able to manage grief within a set period of time, usually a far shorter time than one would think adequate for one's patients" (p. 142). For example, Therapist D (a psychiatrist) had a mild foot infection, but it required prolonged intravenous antibiotics in the hospital. Because he felt well, wanted to work, and had the reassurance of having read my article (Grunebaum 1973), he decided to see his individual patients and his groups in his hospital room.

Working While in Discomfort or Pain

Quite a number of therapists both in the literature and in the interview study indicated that they had worked even though they did not feel entirely well. Silver (1982), an inpatient psychiatrist, described that after an operation for a life-threatening illness her surgeon ordered her to "resume work promptly, seeing anxiety and self-preoccupation as stressful"; so she returned to work, "partly as a therapist, partly as a patient on an occupational therapy assignment" (p. 314).

When I began seeing patients during my hospitalization I was in mild pain but did so because, "I felt mentally alert enough to do so" (Grunebaum 1973, p. 41). Other therapists have reported the same, including the three therapists in the interview sample who worked during the course of their chemotherapy treatment (Morrison, Therapist C, and Therapist E). This was also true for Therapist F, who saw patients for months, while recovering from a serious leg injury. There is no objective way of assessing whether their ability to work was influenced adversely by the discomfort, pain, or fatigue they were experiencing. As far as I could learn they all believed that they were doing competent work and that they were "good enough" therapists.

Therapist E, spoke to me at length about her experience of working while in pain. It had been important to her to work, and she discussed both her intention to work with her clients and the possibility that she might be working with pain. She said she preferred the pain to the feelings of drowsiness and disorientation that analgesic medications produced. She made it clear to her clients that she would not see them if she felt she "could not be entirely present" and that she had no expectations that they "had" to do anything for her, like comfort or support her. Given this contract, she felt able to tell a few clients who asked how she was doing, and who she believed wanted a full answer, that she was "having a hard time," when in fact she was uncomfortable.

Her clients developed a "uniform strategy" to deal with her 9 months of treatment. They would "come in and look me in the eye and ask 'How are you?' I would tell them the truth—often one word: 'fine'—and sometimes they would talk about it for few minutes and sometimes not." It rarely came up at other times in the session, but if it did it was discussed fully.

Other therapists also reported that their patients dealt with having an "impaired therapist" in very similar ways: a brief inquiry followed by a typical psychotherapeutic session. When patients were aware that their therapists were in pain, some of them indicated that they found it difficult to accept help and support from "someone in that situation."

Nothing has been written about therapists who work while in chronic pain, yet given the frequency of conditions such as arthritis this must be quite common. Probably the experience is felt to be too mundane and ordinary to deserve comment. A striking example of chronic illness was related to me by the colleague of a social worker who routinely told her patients that she was on renal dialysis to explain her regular absences and occasional hospitalization. Her orthodox psychoanalytic colleagues decried this openness, but as far as the informant (who was the director of the clinic) could ascertain, her patients continued in effective psychotherapy.

Nature of the Social Network of the Therapist and the Patient

Some patients and therapists have totally separate networks, but others have overlapping ones. It is probably difficult, if not impossible, for a training analyst to keep candidates they are analyzing from learning about their illness when they belong to the same institute. This is true also for patients and therapists from the same hospital and in some communities, as Mazer (1970), who was a psychiatrist on Martha's Vineyard, Massachusetts, described. Given the focus of this chapter, it is of interest that Mazer found it possible to be an effective psychotherapist in a community where both he and the patient were likely to have a lot of information about each other. In addition, the patient and the therapist may have friends in common. As Therapist E (a psychologist and family therapist) stated, "It is essential that patients hear from me, not from my network." Rosner (1986), a psychologist and psychoanalyst, noted that "the ill analyst is not isolated from his patient. Word gets around" (p. 362).

Emotional and Mental State of the Therapist

Without doubt the personal style and character of the therapist are the most important influences on how and what patients will be told about their therapist's illness or injury. The psychologist colleague of the social worker on renal dialysis emphasized the fact that therapists must be comfortable with what they say and do. Like all human beings, therapists have their own personal reactions to illness and injury and yet there is a common core to these feelings. A usual sequence in facing illness often begins with denial, which precedes the diagnosis. This may then be followed by depression and anger. The illness often seems endless and the isolation consequent to it intolerable. Perhaps therapists, engaging as they do in a profession that involves intimate relationships with other human beings, are particularly vulnerable to isolation. I had wondered when I saw patients during my hospitalization whether "perhaps, in fact, I was acting out some fantasy of needing the reassurance and comfort of my patients" (Grunebaum 1973, p. 41). Awareness of these needs is essential for the therapists who continues to work while impaired.

Many authors (Abend [1982] in particular) have described the influence of these feelings on therapists' behavior both in deciding whether to inform the patient and in conducting therapy after the acute illness is over. During this period, the therapist must contend with his or her wishes to be well and to hold to the familiar role of healer; the therapist may not want to admit to the patient that he or she is also a patient, a wounded healer. During my most recent injury episode, I was concerned that a patient of mine who had easy access to my medical records might look at them. I mentioned my wish for privacy to him, and he replied, "Are you worried I'll find out that you're accident prone!" That was precisely what I was worried about.

Clearly, each therapist must assess the state of his or her own feelings on returning to work and act accordingly using the same clinical judgment used in regard to other clinical issues. The issue of the denial of illness is a thorny one. Schwartz (1987), a psychoanalyst, commented that "the collusive denial by one's treating medical doctors of the emotional impact of one's illness . . . and their exhortations to forget the past can interfere with meaningful self-analytic resolution of the unconscious impact of the illness" (p. 666). However, denial may be useful. Based on years of experience consulting with patients undergoing cardiac bypass surgery, Blacher (personal communication, November 1989), a Boston psychoanalyst, found that psychiatrists in particular have to be encouraged and supported in their denial, as denial correlates with favorable outcome. Reiss et al. (1986), for example, found that family denial promotes longevity in patients undergoing renal dialysis. Perhaps there is a certain amount of useful denial of our mortality that permits us to take pleasure in life, even in the face of our knowledge of our mortality, whereas, in contrast, denial of our particular affective states may impede us in our understanding of ourselves and thus of our patients.

WHAT TO TELL PATIENTS

It is significant that all the therapists I interviewed and, indeed, all therapists in the literature (including Abend [1982], who suggested that therapists should not tell their patients) did in fact tell most of their patients about their illness or injury. They dealt with their illness in ways that were far more similar than different. Each told patients something about the facts of the illness, prepared them for absences when possible, and told some of what had happened afterward. This was particularly true if absences were prolonged or there were obvious sequelae of the illness. Each endeavored to be honest and straightforward, and each individualized what they told their patients and answered questions when asked. On the other hand, several therapists indicated to me that they believed their patients did not know about their major illness or surgery (despite the fact that I, who was only very peripherally involved with them, knew about it). It must be emphasized that a delicate balance exists between revealing too much (and thus burdening the patient) and being insufficiently open or deceptive. Clinical decisions must be made precisely at a time when the therapist is convalescing and is less able to make these judgments wisely. This is an instance in which consultation with a trusted colleague may be invaluable.

The only exception to a straightforward approach was that used by Lindner (1984), who initially communicated a "fabrication" to explain his sudden absence, which occurred 1 week before an already announced vacation. He had his secretary inform his patients that a family emergency had arisen necessitating his leaving 1 week earlier than anticipated. When it became clear that he required surgery, he wrote his patients informing them of the factual details of his illness and of his anticipated return. He did not, however, describe the effects, if any, of the discrepancy between these two explanations. A different example is that of Morrison (1990), who decided she would "respond honestly to those who wanted to know, would not initiate any self disclosures, and above all would listen" (p. 234).

An understanding of how much the therapist can comfortably reveal must take into account character. There are individuals who are inclined to be open about their personal experiences and those who value privacy more. Some therapists share much with their friends and colleagues and others share more sparingly. In addition, it must be expected that therapists will adapt to a diagnosis with varying degrees of speed and acceptance. Therapist G (a psychoanalyst), who acquired a hearing aid, related that, "Perhaps at first I was proud that I had gone and gotten it, proud of my new toy, and a little bit exhibitionistic." Later he found "it more of a handicap and nuisance and downplayed it." The therapist's own reaction to illness and injury clearly changes over time. We cannot expect that we can automatically do what is best for our patients, know what we will say, or know how honest to be when the situation makes us anxious ourselves.

The diversity of reasons therapists gave for telling their patients the truth was striking. At this point, it is useful to reemphasize that regardless of what patients are told or not told, many of them will find out the truth. Some therapists stated simply that they believed therapists should be honest with their patients. For instance, Therapist H (a training analyst) said, "Have you ever known anyone who was harmed by the truth?" Another therapist indicated that a belief in "second-order cybernetics" was the intellectual underpinning for telling her patients the truth. Therapist E said that she believed the therapist was a collaborator in the therapeutic process, not an observer of it: "Being intensely present is central to my therapy. I have to be honest to maintain my authenticity and to maintain my part of the authenticity of the relationship. Not sharing something that is so central a part of my on-going moment-to-moment experiences, and that does have an impact on clients in terms of scheduling, appearance, etc., feels like a kind of dishonesty that I would not want to introduce into my work."

My own reasoning for telling my patients the truth was my belief that the therapist is a model for identification as a "person who attempts to face and deal with himself, his problems and life—not someone without problems either internal or external . . . expecting the utmost in candor from my patients, I could ask no less of myself, and I told my patients about my injury when I called them" (Grunebaum 1973, p. 41).

A major reason that many therapists gave for telling the truth was their own personal experiences with therapists who had concealed their illness from patients. Therapist A related, "I had seen what happened when L., who was a teacher I admired, was ill and died not having told his patients and resolved to act differently. I, therefore, told them about my cardiac bypass operation."

A friend (an analyst) told me that his training analyst had had a stroke and that when she returned and resumed her practice she told him she had injured her back. His colleagues were incredulous that he did not know what had really happened. Therapist H reported that he was very troubled that none of the patients of another analyst had been told that he was terminally ill and described how betrayed and deceived the patients felt. Both of these therapists emphasized very specifically that they had been influenced by these experiences early in their careers. Finally, Morrison (1990) summed up this issue saying, "Over the years I have known many instances in which patients were abandoned by ill or dying therapists, therapists who denied the gravity of their own illness or impending death, and did not attempt to say goodbye or help their patients connect with another therapist" (p.228).

The validity of these observations is supported by research done by Dattner (1985), who found that patients who were kept in the dark about the terminal illness of their therapist felt painfully deceived and very guilty about knowing what they were not supposed to know. More recently, Tallmer (1989) interviewed 15 psychoanalytic candidates whose training analyst had died. She concluded that although it has been suggested that there are treatment situations in which a discussion of the analyst's actual impending death would be harmful, to avoid the subject may produce more long-lasting, deleterious effects and an important, in vivo opportunity for an honest, authentic, real way of relating to another may be missed.

It seems to me that therapists who do not tell their patients about serious illnesses are engaging in a denial and arrogating to themselves the inappropriate position of concealing important information. For example, Schwartz (1987) had major surgery for a large mass of unknown origin in his right chest cavity. The mass turned out to be benign and he recovered completely. He did not tell his patients anything except that he had a medical problem that had been taken care of and was not expected to recur. On the other hand, Schwartz also stated, "as analysand, I felt abandoned and profoundly shaken by my analyst's repeated hospitalizations and ultimately his sudden death" (p. 671). Despite his own experience, Schwartz apparently believed that his future was secure and certain, but perhaps he, like most of us, was engaging in necessary denial. Moreover, a study of older analysts by Tallmer (1989) suggested that analysts can be as adroit as (or perhaps even more adroit than) anyone else in resisting the emergence of uncomfortable affect, for less than one half of the 94 analysts in her study had discussed the possibility of their eventual death with patients.

Although therapists believe that they should tell their patients about their illness, it appears that this may require some degree of optimism about the outcome. Some therapists with a recurrence of a malignancy may find it impossible to share this with their patients. Their own needs for privacy conflict with their belief in telling the truth. And perhaps they do not want to burden their patients.

The clearest exposition of the reasons for not telling patients about one's illness is that by Abend (1982), who almost uniquely espouses this position. Before examining Abend's reasoning, it is interesting to note that Schwartz (1987) felt that, "What is perhaps most evocative about Abend's paper is that throughout it, he tells us nothing about his illness. We, the readers, are left to experience along with his patients the same insisted-upon vacuum of information, as well as the scopophilic fantasies it gives rise to. . . . Equally telling is the realization that knowing the facts of Abend's illness is irrelevant to comprehending his thesis" (p. 668).

For Abend (1982), the specifics of a diagnosis (including what immediate and enduring effects the illness might have on the analyst) did not influence his conclusion that one should say nothing to patients. Abend noted that the decision of what to tell the patient is being made precisely when the therapist is influenced by powerful countertransferences and, therefore, is least able to make the decision uninfluenced by powerful countertransference and probably tells the patient out of a need to "subserve unconscious needs." Van Dam (1987), a Los Angeles psychoanalyst, agreed with Abend that saying nothing was best. In their opinion, to say anything at all will inevitably involve distortions caused by the therapist's post-illness countertransference, because, as Schwartz (1987) noted in summarizing Abend, "clinical experience at other times invariably attests to the advantage of not informing patients of the details of one's life, the same is true after an illness" (p. 668).

One wonders what Schwartz (1987) meant by "details." Were my sling and external fixator, Dewald's eye-patch (1982), and Morrison's loss of hair (1990) "details," or were they such obdurate realities that some explanation had to be given. Therapist G, for instance, reported that several of his patients were grateful to him for wearing a hearing aid. He, of course, did not have to explain what the device was. Yet, each of these evidences of disability served as a stimulus for fantasies, each had transference implications, and none seemed to interfere with the progress of therapy.

There are also patients who do not notice major changes in the appearance of the therapist. This situation poses a difficult clinical dilemma because the therapist must decide whether to bring the subject up for discussion. For example, Morrison (1990) reported that some of her patients did not notice marked changes, such as the appearance of her wig. (She viewed this "as a manifestation of self-absorption and reflection of narcissism" [p. 234].) In such instances, the therapist can only use clinical judgment about whether or not to bring the subject up with the patient. Further, even when the therapist is being honest and open, some patients will deny the illness and the changes in the therapist's appearance and/or feel betrayed and abandoned.

Therapists will be misguided and act defensively if they expect that giving patients information will modulate their anger or increase their sympathy. Rosner (1986) suggested the opposite, that the more information the patient has, the greater the hostility will be that the therapist must contend with. In their discussion about sharing the death of a loved one with patients, Givelber and Simon (1981) commented, "It is unlikely that the recently bereaved therapist can in anticipation know the best strategy for each patient and perfectly negotiate various therapeutic snares" (p. 145). It is my impression, however, that patients will be both sympathetic and angry, influenced most by the extent to which the event interferes with their treatment. This issue requires further exploration.

Although Abend's article (1982) illustrated one extreme of the continuum of therapist anonymity, he also described his discussions with colleagues: "Almost to a man [sic], they had arrived at something equivalent to Dewald's solution. . . . There apparently exists a sort of common-sense consensus . . ." (p. 371) to tell patients something about the facts. What is perhaps most remarkable about Abend, himself, is that despite his resolve not to say anything to his patients, "within three days. . . I found equally compelling reasons to tell all but two of my analytic patients something factual about my illness" (p. 374). As far as one can judge from Abend's article, none of his patients suffered as a consequence of his telling them. At this juncture, it is important to reiterate that not only had all of the therapists I interviewed told their patients something about their illness, they all believed that it had not adversely influenced the course of the psychotherapy.

Reactions of Patients to the
Therapist's Illness or Injury

All the therapists (in both the literature and the interviews) reported that, as expected, their patients responded to their illness or injury in terms of the relationship between them and that their own psychodynamics and the characteristics of the relationship played a major role in that response. Therapist I (a young woman resident), who had to be out for 2 weeks to have an operation on her wrist, returned to work with a cast on her forearm. Different patients reacted quite differently: with anger at her for being away, "I can't even look at your cast. . . . I feel completely abandoned"; with anger for having to be sorry for her, "I dreamt you were sick and I had to take care of you, which I resented"; with concern that she would now not attend to their problems; and with anxiety that they might lose her.

A useful example of the response of a quite disturbed patient was reported by Silver (1982). She related that a 23-year-old chronically borderline psychotic woman first sent her a get-well card in the hospital and later a book, *For Colored Girls Who Have Considered Suicide When The Rainbow Is Enuf* (Shange 1975). When Silver returned to work, the patient asked, "'Can I hug you?' I said 'Yes' and we hugged and cried" (p. 371). This case illustrates a particularly important dynamic of many patients, who, as Silver stated, are "individuals who have tried but failed to be therapists to troubled family members" (p. 322).

It is also true, as Singer (1971) and I (Grunebaum 1973) have noted, that there are few, if any, opportunities for patients to be caring of their therapists. Singer, an existential psychoanalyst, described telling his patients of his wife's serious illness and learned that "the capacity to rise to the occasion when compassion and helpfulness are called for is part and parcel of the makeup of all human beings. Importantly, in no single instance did my disclosure have any ill effects; on the contrary, the insights, memories, and heightened awareness which followed my self-disclosure proved remarkable and I have the deep conviction that my frankness accelerated the therapeutic process in several instances" (p. 41). Likewise, Silver (1982) noted that she experienced certain patients as "constructive loving forces" in her life. Both Singer and Silver found their patients supportive and helpful and that this afforded the patient an opportunity to show a different aspect of themselves to the therapist. As I indicated above, this was also true with my patients.

Exploring what it means for the patient to care for the therapist—to show this side of his or her personality—may be as important as studying how he or she experiences the therapist's caring for them. Yet it is also true that, as Therapist C observed, "the patient cannot have to treat you"; in other words, the therapist bears the ultimate responsibility for the therapy. Several therapists indicated during the interviews that their patients had given them useful advice. For instance, Therapist B related that a patient, who was an internist, told him not to have a by-pass and suggested that he consult a well-known expert. He said of his patient, "I assumed that I was taking good care of him and that he would do the same for me."

Are there any generalizations about how one should approach patients? Dewald (1982) tailored his approach to the needs of each patient according to his best clinical judgment at the time. On the other hand, Abend (1982) felt that "the very clinical judgement relied on . . . is exactly what is under pressure from the countertransference [and] is less likely to be objective and reliable" (p. 370). Of course this is equally true for the decision to reveal nothing. However, most authors agree that sicker patients should be told more factual information and healthier ones less, that patients in psychotherapy should receive more information and those in analysis less, and that those earlier in treatment may need more information than those who have been in treatment longer.

Thus far this discussion has focused on what the therapist should say to the patient. It may be useful at this point to emphasize that not telling the patient is not a neutral action. Rather, as Rosner (1986) emphasized, "Action is being taken by the analyst towards the patient . . . who may react . . . to the act of withholding information" (p. 361). This may lead the patient to feel "dismissed, shut out, unimportant, treated like a child," and so on (p. 361). Rosner concluded, "Thus in the service of maintaining neutrality, in avoiding the risk of introducing countertransferential distortions, and in supporting an open field for unconscious interplay and transference distortions by maintaining a nonfactual, nonrevelatory position, one runs a counter risk of introducing real issues of exclusion, abandonment, and rejection" (p. 362).

The ill or injured therapist may be usefully compared with the pregnant therapist (see Chapter 7). An obvious difference is that pregnancy is usually a welcome event to the therapist. In both cases, however, a real event intrudes into the therapy. Some patients will notice and comment early and others only after the pregnancy is quite advanced. Balsam, a psychoanalyst and one of the first to write about this subject, commented that if a patient does not say anything about a pregnancy, she would bring it up with them (R. Balsam, personal communication, June 1991). This is precisely what Dewald (1982) did with a patient who "resumed analysis with no mention whatsoever of the separation" due to his serious illness (p. 365). Perhaps the most important issue noted in the literature on the pregnant therapist is that no one believes that seeing a therapist who becomes pregnant is harmful to most patients.

However, some patients may find this change in the therapist difficult to tolerate and all patients will have feelings, thoughts, and fantasies about it.

Just as some patients will find a therapist's pregnancy intolerable, so too will some find discussing their therapist's illness or injury intolerable. Regardless of what one does, some patients will terminate treatment. For example, one of Morrison's patients had a previous therapist, whom he had just come to trust, who died, leaving him feeling utter and total abandonment (Morrison 1990). He could not tolerate having another therapist with cancer and terminated. On the other hand, Weinberg (1988), an analyst, found that very few of her patients dropped out. She commented, "After all, if I could deal with my real-life events maybe they could deal with the anxieties and concerns of dealing with their own" (p. 459).

It does not appear that the ill or injured therapist can follow any course that will not lead to a few patients terminating therapy, while most continue in treatment. However, as emphasized earlier, the harmful effects of the therapist's death for which the patient could have been prepared and was not are simply too great.

Are the Therapist's Actions an Important Model for the Patient?

Another way of looking at the issues facing therapists is by clarifying the various ways that therapists influence patients. Because therapy is a type of learning, it is important to be aware that, as Chasin and I (see Grunebaum and Chasin 1982) have discussed, all theories of learning can be placed under one of three major rubrics. The one that is most emphasized in the therapy literature, particularly the psychoanalytic literature, is that of gaining insight and understanding. Therapy, however, also offers opportunities for identification and imitation as well as for conditioning and behavioral reinforcement. Although the therapist may attempt to maximize one of these methods of learning, the patient may learn in another. For instance, some patients may experience the therapist's comments as behavioral reinforcement, without attending to the content of the comments. Finally, it must be emphasized that the therapist cannot act in a way that prevents learning in all of these modes. Regardless of how invisible and neutral the therapist attempts to be, the patient can and often will identify with them, perhaps becoming more neutral, detached, and invisible in their own life.

If patients tend to identify with their therapists, what sort of person the therapist is, what kind of a life he or she lives, and how he or she faces illness, injury, and death are of utmost moment. As Morrison

(1990) noted, "There may also be some real therapeutic advantage for the patient in the therapist's example of the capacity to bear ambiguity, or to face the unbearable" (p. 249). Returning to the experience of Caron, one of his patients said, "If this man can go on living in spite of his illness, then I too can try to do something about my own life" (Meloche 1984, p.333). Finally, Goldberg (1984), a psychiatric social worker, concluded an article saying, "In those instances when I shared openly the nature of my [fatal] illness and my reactions to it, an intimacy developed far surpassing anything I had experienced previously in my work. People grasped the humanness of the situation and banded together to lend help and support to one another and to me in performing the hard task of saying good-bye" (p. 296). However, we cannot expect that therapists should face death in ways that demand more of them than we do of others. As Morrison (1990) noted, "We know that reactions to major life events are idiosyncratic, at the same time that they hold universals. It may not be humanly possible to handle a frightening illness, a threat to own's life in a way that is optimal and ideal for patients. We cannot prepare for all eventualities" (p. 249).

Nonetheless, I would suggest that it is the integrity and dedication of the therapist to the welfare of his or her patients that is crucial. This may be related to what Schwartz (1987) was describing when he referred to the "continued intactness of the analytic field." But the intactness of that field, as we have seen, depends on its being intact, and when the therapist is ill or injured the field is no longer intact. Indeed, we may question the very concept of "intactness" in human relationships; perhaps, "good enough" is a more realistic goal.

Working While Adversely Influenced by Illness or Injury

Unfortunately, because we are not omnipotent, the therapeutic relationship may at times be influenced or impaired because of events in the our lives. Among such events are injury, illness, pregnancy, and deaths in the family. To quote Silver (1982), "If the ideal therapist serves as a secure container for the projected affects of the patient, I guiltily thought of myself as more a colander or saturated sponge than a container" (p. 314). Silver also reported the importance to her of working in a particularly holding environment at Chestnut Lodge. Dewald (1982) noted that "not only is there a heightened susceptibility to fatigue, but there is difficulty in returning to an optimal analytic posture ... and there persists a degree of self-absorption and continued preoccupation with the residues of the illness" (p. 354). Further, Morrison (1990) commented that at a certain point in the course of her cancer when the prognosis seemed particularly bad, "[I was] depressed anyway, and was less 'there' for my patients. The silence of my disease was, at this time, deafening for me" (p.241). And Therapist A, who had the coronary bypass with complications, returned to work, "looking like the wrath of God, but feeling blessed that I had been given extra-time." On the whole, however, little has been written about the therapist who returns to work not fully recovered.

What effect does a therapist's working while in pain or discomfort or depressed have on the patient? Feeling rather uncomfortable about undertaking this inquiry, I asked a few patients recently who had seen me during my shoulder fracture if they had been aware I was in pain and what effect this had on their therapy. They indicated that they had most certainly been aware of my pain and stated in one way or another that, "I'm here to work on my problems and I intend to do so." I am impressed in retrospect that all of my patients continued in treatment with me and seemed to make progress satisfactory to both them and to me. Rather similar experiences were related by Therapist J (a social worker), who had had a rather prolonged and severe neurotic depression. Probably most patients were aware of her depression; about half commented or asked questions about her mood, and none terminated. She believed that she was a good therapist during this period and, in fact, found her work pleasurable and satisfying while taking little pleasure in anything else.

Silver (1982) also commented on the patients she was working with who were "striving to work with me, working to get through the sessions, then to get something from them, then to reestablish the former equilibrium . . . to rebuild the holding environment" (p. 324). She was grateful to these patients and confident they knew this. Silver also described the uncertainties of her work during this period. This uncertainty was also true for me and perhaps for other therapists working when not at their best. The assured therapist undoubtedly sets a different example of how to live life than does the one who experiences and even acknowledges uncertainty. Indeed, acknowledging uncertainty is a kind of assurance in an uncertain world.

The recovering, but not fully recovered therapist will be tired, worried, in pain, and/or weak. Therapist J reported her anger at her analyst for his refusal to acknowledge his back pain of which she was aware from the way he shifted in his chair and his awkward posture when arising. She commented that all he would need to have done was say "Yes, my back hurts today," and been willing to have her discuss her feelings about this. His attitude seemed to reflect his own feelings of being intruded on and exposed and precluded open exploration.

Given that patients are able to deal successfully with many exigencies in their therapist's lives, it may be worth considering whether they should be informed of other major events in the therapist's life that may alter the therapeutic climate. Although the therapist may attempt to "manage" the feelings engendered on his or her own, this attempt can probably never be entirely successful. Insofar as the therapist's life experiences enter the therapy it may be important that the patient be made aware that some changes in the therapeutic climate are not his or her responsibility. Issues concerning the therapist's right to appropriate privacy and undue impingement during therapy deserve serious consideration when issues of therapist openness are being considered.

The effects of these states of mind and body are not all bad; as Morrison (1990) commented, "There has also been another side: an energizing, a greater attunement to my patients, a sense of myself as courageous and as physically and emotionally strong, an experiencing of this siege as providing a strangely useful opportunity. . . . I often felt that I was able to listen with a 'fourth' ear, particularly for issues of loss and meaning around my absences" (p. 229).

On the other hand, the chronically ill therapist faces a difficult road. Therapist K (a psychiatrist-psychoanalyst) had chronic diabetes and slowly evolving complications. He spoke of his uncertain recent memory, his need at times to keep his mouth shut lest he make an error, and his telling some of his patients he was on medication when he nodded off during therapy. He said, "Patients don't know, I believe, but I do." He said he wondered how long he would be able to practice. Yet both nodding off and forgetting are common in middle age, if not, indeed, during all of life.

In addition, we can never be sure if the patient is not responding to clues about us that arise in associations that they do not feel free to inquire about. An example of such a situation occurred recently in a group psychotherapy session I was leading. I had had minor facial surgery earlier that week for what turned out to be a small basal cell cancer beside my nose. The stitches and gauze were hardly noticeable, but the group inquired what had happened. I told them that I had minor surgery the previous day. The group then began a long discussion that gradually centered on the subject of parental trustworthiness and honesty. I wondered out loud if this was a question they also had about me. They indicated it was and that they felt I had not given them a complete answer to their questions about what had happened. I then told them the results of the biopsy, and they went on to discuss the importance of knowing the truth. Group psychotherapy is a setting rather different from individual psychotherapy. As Goldberg (1984) noted, "What enabled them [her group] to inquire was the mutual support and encouragement they gave and continue to give one another, in the expression of their anxieties and fantasies" (p. 290). She noted that the "reaction of this group, as well as each stage that has followed, has been paralleled in my work with individuals" (p. 291).

Insofar as one views the patient as an equal adult participant in the treatment and the treatment as an object relationship, one will believe that "much of what the patient feels may be an accurate perception of change resulting from the illness" (Dewald 1982, p. 307). As Morrison (1990) pointed out, "For many a patient, the therapist's refusal to acknowledge the patient's awareness of the therapist's vulnerability becomes a repetition of past, deleterious experience [of] efforts to cloak, hide, or forbid talk about 'bad' events in the name of protection, but almost always resulting in confusion" (p. 248). The single most moving example of the patient's response to a change in the therapist is described by Chernin (1976) who quoted Berlin's experience with a non-verbal psychotic child: "The first words of the psychotic child were in response to the therapist becoming acutely ill in the playroom. She sat with the therapist until he felt better, repeatedly saying, 'Poor Dr. Berlin,' her first speech, as she stroked his head" (p. 1328).

CONCLUSIONS

The therapist is a participant in the treatment, and how he or she deals with the illness will have a major role in determining the patient's responses. As Anna Freud stated, "We should leave room for the realization that the analyst and the patient are also two real people, of equal adult status, in a real personal relationship to each other" (see Rosner 1986, p. 369).

Distinguishing between fantasy and reality, between accurate perception and transference distortion, is a task that the therapist and the patient can and, I believe, should share. For this to happen the patient must have available the necessary information to make that distinction.

It should be evident by now that I believe, based on both a review of the literature and an interview study of therapists, that one should tell the patient the truth about serious illnesses and injuries. This is also true for minor ones that have visible sequelae. The therapist must endeavor to become comfortable with being honest about his or her impairment and discuss it with the patient in a way that opens rather than closes down therapeutic conversation. Clearly, what is said must be individualized to meet the particular character and style of each patient and the state of the relationship with the therapist.

That most therapists in the literature and the interviews (save for a few psychoanalysts) agreed about the appropriate course of action is itself an interesting fact. These therapists included psychiatrists, psychologists, and social workers, who worked with different populations in different settings and espoused different theories, but they agreed on the appropriate course of action. The same kind of agreement was noted by Jonsen and Toulmin (1988). Based on their experience in the National Commission for the Protection of Human Subjects of Biomedical and Behavioral Research, they reported that members of the commission were largely in agreement about their specific practical conclusions, but not about why they agreed. The authors suggested that the commission "shared a perception of what was specifically at stake in particular kinds of human situations" (p. 18). But why should this be so?

I believe the reason is that therapists who base their conclusions on theory—a particular reading of psychoanalytic theory—come to one conclusion that, interestingly, they have difficulty following. They seem to believe that they can be an observer of the therapy, rather than a participant in it. However, the vast majority of therapists view the situation of the ill or injured therapist from the perspective of the actual relationship in which two human beings are working together. Viewed in this way (as a human situation, a human predicament), the natural conclusion is to tell the truth, to face the facts, and as best as humanly possible to deal with them realistically, caringly, therapeutically, and (because illness or injury is a tragic event) often painfully.

A POSTSCRIPT ON ETHICS

In concluding this chapter, I would like to set the issues of telling patients an appropriate amount of information about an illness or injury in a larger perspective and discuss them from an ethical point of view. Most of what I have discussed until this point has dealt with the therapist-patient relationship in factual and dynamic terms. There is, however, also an ethical basis to this relationship as, indeed, there is to all relationships. I believe we should think about the ethics of therapy in the broadest possible way in terms of the effects of the whole of the therapeutic relationship on the patient.

The conflict that therapists experience when they confront discussing their own impairment with a patient is between their adherence to two different ethical conceptions. On the one hand, they see themselves as attempting to help the patient in gaining insight and changing, while they remain constant in their devotion to a theory of psychotherapy.

Their ethic is one of adherence to the value of constancy and devotion to their role of self-denial and neutrality. They endeavor to make no personal or emotional demands of the patient. The roots of this conception of ethics are in Plato who believed that the good life required the pursuit of a single transcendent value: in his case, justice. This value was seen as above and beyond ordinary human commitments. On the other hand, the therapist can also see himself or herself as a human being—one whose manner of facing life can be a model to the patient—and as a person having knowledge and wisdom about human relationships, what Aristotle (Gould 1975) called *phronesis*. The therapist must then be willing to face his or her own weaknesses and impairments and acknowledge them to the patient. To paraphrase the Nussbaum (1986) quote at the beginning of this chapter, human excellence involves, in part, human vulnerability. This ethical belief has its roots in Aristotle, who felt that ethics must take into account the many goods that make for a full human life.

I believe that decisions about the therapeutic endeavor remain matters of practical wisdom rather than being derivable from theory. Aristotle noted that in areas of human endeavor that demand practical wisdom (phronesis) we should not seek the same degree of certainty we do in science. Philosophers have recently been interested in "casuistry," which is seen as deriving ethical principles from the bottom up (from cases), rather than from the top down, which emphasizes theory, deduction, and the quest for moral certainty (Jonsen and Toulmin 1988). In this view, which I share, virtue may lie in accepting a degree of uncertainty and fallibility rather than yielding to the desire for rigid rules.

In deciding what to tell patients one can either live up to the ideals of a good human relationship or betray it. This is the reason why patients who have not been informed of their therapist's terminal illness, when this was possible, feel so betrayed. They have been betrayed, either because of the therapist's own needs or because the therapist dealt with the situation in a technical or theoretically correct way with regard for the human relationship. And this is also why patients, who can share their therapist's illness (even terminal illness), who work together in therapy, and who grieve together, do well. In a less dramatic way, therapists who validate what their patients observe can do effective psychotherapy while pregnant, while grief-stricken, and while suffering the pains and discomforts of illness and injury. Beyond our obligations to our patients as their therapist with personal and technical skills, we have an ethical obligation to be worthy of their trust in us as fellow human beings. Being a "good therapist" is not separable from being a good person.

Epilogue

Since I first completed this chapter, a colleague and good friend of mine has suffered the loss of her analyst. He had been extraordinarily helpful and caring, and she was devoted to him. She saw him following surgery for cancer, but when a recurrence led to his terminal illness, she was discouraged from attempting to see or call him. She felt that she had been unable to say goodbye. In addition, she found that during the service after his death, no mention was made of his patients or their thoughts and feelings about this man who had spent so much of his life devoted to them.

This experience makes tragically clear that we must take into account, somehow, that not only our family and friends suffer a grievous loss when we die, our patients do also (these issues are addressed in more detail in Chapter 3). We cannot invite and foster intimate and caring relationships with our patients and then think that our death will be easily dealt with by them. We should endeavor to make some place in the services and funeral for their grief and perhaps even for their words. It seems too much to ask that bereaved families and friends should take outsiders into account at the time of such a loss. Rather, it would seem our responsibility to address this consequence of the kind of human relationships we have with our patients. Although our fellow professionals do the same kind of work we do, it is our patients who are truly our colleagues in working together at a shared task.

References

Abend SM: Serious illness in the analyst: countertransference considerations. J Am Psychoanal Assoc 30:365–379, 1982

Chernin P: Illness in a therapist: loss of omnipotence. Arch Gen Psychiatry 33:1327–1328, 1976

Deutsch CJ: A survey of therapists' personal problems and treatment. Professional Psychology: Research and Practice 16:305–315, 1985

Dattner R: The death of an analyst: theoretical and clinical issues. Panel conducted at the annual meeting of the Division of Psychoanalysis, American Psychological Association, New York, April 1985

Dewald P: Serious illness in the analyst: transference, countertransference, and reality responses. J Am Psychoanal Assoc 30:347–363, 1982

Givelber F, Simon B: A death in the life of a therapist and its impact on the therapy. Psychiatry 44:141–149, 1981

Goldberg F: Personal observations of a therapist with a life-threatening illness. Int J Group Psychother 34:289–296, 1984

Gould GP (ed): Aristotle's Nichomachean Ethics: Book II. Translated by Rackham H. Cambridge, MA, Harvard University Press, 1975

Grunebaum H: Psychotherapy during the therapist's recovery from an injury. Psychiatric Opinion, October:39–42, 1973

Grunebaum H, Chasin R: Thinking like a family therapist. Journal of Marital and Family Therapy 8:403–416, 1982

Guy JD, Souder JK: Impact of therapists' illness or accident on psychotherapeutic practice: review and discussion. Professional Psychology: Research and Practice 17:509–513, 1986

Hannett F: Transference reactions to an event in the life of the analyst. Psychoanal Rev 36:69–81, 1949

Jonsen AR, Toulmin S: The Abuse of Casuistry: A History of Moral Reasoning. Berkeley, CA, University of California Press, 1988

Morrison AL: Doing psychotherapy while living with a life-threatening illness, in Illness in the Analyst. Edited by Schwartz HS, Silver AL. Madison, CT, International Universities Press, 1990, pp 227–250

Lindner H: Therapist and patient reactions to life-threatening crises in the therapist's life. Psychotherapy in Private Practice 2(4):73–78, 1984

Mazer M: The therapist in the community, in The Practice of Community Mental Health. Edited by Grunebaum H. Boston, MA, Little, Brown, 1970, pp 663–683

Meloche M: The patient and the dying psychiatrist. Can J Psychiatry 29:330–334, 1984

Nussbaum M: The Fragility of Goodness: Luck and Ethics in Greek Tragedy and Philosophy. Cambridge, England, Cambridge University Press, 1986

Oesterheld JR, Buckman D: Four aspects of therapists' acute illness and injury that trigger transference reactions, in Psychotherapy in Private Practice, Vol 7. Binghamton, NY, Haworth Press, 1989, pp 41–53

Reiss D, Gonzalez S, Kramer N: Family process, chronic illness, and death: on the weakness of strong bonds. Arch Gen Psychiatry 43:795–804, 1986

Rosner S: The seriously ill or dying analyst and the limits of neutrality. Psychoanalytic Psychology 3:357–371, 1986

Schwartz HJ: Illness in the doctor: implications for the psychoanalytic process. J Am Psychoanal Assoc 35:657–692, 1987

Shange N: For Colored Girls Who Have Considered Suicide When the Rainbow Is Enuf. New York, Macmillan, 1975

Silver AL: Resuming the work with a life-threatening illness. Contemporary Psychoanalysis 18:314–326, 1982

Singer E: The patient aids the analyst: some clinical and theoretical observations, in The Name of Life. Edited by Landis B, Tauber E. New York, Holt, Rinehart & Winston, 1971

Tallmer M: The death of an analyst. Psychoanal Rev 76:529–542, 1989

van Dam H: Countertransference during an analyst's brief illness. J Am Psychoanal Assoc 35:647–655, 1987

Weinberg H: Illness and the working analyst. Reprinted in Contemporary Psychoanalysis 24:452–461, 1988

Weissman MM, Merikangas KR, Boyd JH: Epidemiology of affective disorders (Chapter 60), in Psychiatry. Edited by Michaels R. Philadelphia, PA, JB Lippincott, 1989

Chapter 3

The Aging and Dying Psychotherapist: Death and Illness in the Life of the Aging Psychotherapist

Alex H. Kaplan, M.D.

As the psychotherapist ages, there are many factors intimately related to the aging process that influence what goes on within the treatment process. In this chapter I focus on the significance of the positive and negative effects that the aging process, death and illness in the life of the aging psychotherapist, and the dying psychotherapist have on the psychotherapeutic process.

THE AGING PSYCHOTHERAPIST

Defining Aging

During the process of psychotherapy it is inevitable that the psychotherapist will age and therefore be in the process of dying. Yet publications evaluating the effects of the normal aging process on the psychotherapeutic process have only recently begun to appear in our literature. It might be helpful to define *aging*. Birren (1988) defined it as "the transformation of the human organism after the age of maturity—that is, optimum age of reproduction—so that the possibility of survival constantly decreases and there are regular transformations in appearance, behavior, experience and social roles" (p. 159).

We are all aware that as they age, some psychotherapists continue to mature and become more creative, thereby becoming better psychotherapists and educators. On the other hand, some regress as they age, becoming more rigid, inflexible, more dependent and depressed, and unable to deal with the disturbing feelings in their patients, as well as bringing increasing contaminants to their psychotherapy with marked countertransference difficulties. In the aging process, there is more frequently an earlier deterioration of the body than of the mind. Visual, auditory, and motor difficulties and cardiac problems are frequently present changes that need to be accepted and accommodated to by the therapist as well as by the patient. As Eissler (1977) noted, "The aura of the aging psychotherapist in the treatment room significantly modifies the analytic process" (p. 140).

However, some of the most creative accomplishments of artists, writers, musicians, and other professionals, including psychotherapists, have occurred late in their lives even though many of them had a variety of physical disorders associated with aging. Freud is only one of many similar creative persons who actively introduced new concepts in psychoanalysis late in his life, despite serious throat cancer and difficulties in talking. Freud saw patients until several weeks before his death, but there is no evidence he ever discussed the effects of his long involvement with his throat cancer and impending death on his psychotherapeutic endeavors, considerable as those effects must have been (Halpert 1982).

Literature Review

K. R. Eissler (1977) was the first psychoanalyst to discuss in great detail the positive and negative effects of aging on the psychoanalytic process. He pointed out that an earlier analysis does not protect the aging analyst against psychopathological reactions. As they age, some analysts become rigid, compulsive, and depressed. Others may expect too much admiration from their patients. As they age, some analysts become more dependent on their analysands and the analytic process to protect them from their fear of death.

On the other hand, some analysts may become less rigid, and more open and assertive with the development of a more vigorous psychoanalytic process. Eissler urged that aging analysts counsel their patient on what to do or who to turn to in the event of their deaths. Because older psychoanalysts are more likely to die, Eissler felt such action was fully justified. Of course tact and timing are important, as is analyzing the patient's reactions at the time these questions come up. Eissler's other significant conclusion related to the slowly dying psychoanalyst. He suggested that, under such circumstances, heroic posturing by the analyst was not beneficial to the patient. He felt that it was better to discuss the reality of the situation with the patient, continue the analysis for a period so the patient would have time to express his or her feelings and concerns over the inevitable separation and loss, and then transfer the patient to a colleague as soon as the initial reactions have been analytically discussed. Finally, Eissler also felt that it was extremely important for the patient to continue treatment with another analyst while the previous one was still alive.

Additional Data

With the paucity of information about the effects of the aging process on the therapeutic process, I gathered additional information from informal discussions with colleagues and my own experiences. Most of these colleagues were age 65 years or older, still in active practice, and without serious physical disorders. One analyst remarked that earlier in his career he had been more reclusive and reserved, especially with his analysands. As he aged, though, he became more open, not only because he wrote more and gave more talks but because he felt less inhibited about expressing his thoughts and feelings. As a result, his analysands came to know more about him personally than before. But more importantly his analyses were more vigorous, including the transferences that developed. These positive aspects of the aging process are not uncommon.

Another aspect of the aging process relates to the effects that therapists' absences have on patients. As therapists get older, patients may more frequently misconstrue an occasional absence as related to an illness that might lead to separation or loss (see Chapter 4). Thus some therapists tell their patients each January of their coming meetings during the year. But this procedure may have the effect of muting the transference and could be a detriment to therapy, preventing the working through of feelings related to separation and loss.

Countertransference and Transference Reactions

The character of the therapeutic process may change considerably when the therapist is aging because the transference reactions that patients develop are not those to a parent figure but to a grandparent figure. For this reason it becomes more difficult for the patients to express sexual feelings or fantasies because they may feel it is "more disgusting" to mention such feelings to a grandparent figure. But in other situations some patients with sexual concerns may find expressing these concerns to an aging therapist less frightening because he or she is "safer." The same might be true of the expression of aggressive feelings that develop in negative phases of treatment because of the fear that expressing such feelings would be overwhelming and destructive to an aging therapist. One hysterical female patient with repressed anger toward her grandfatherly therapist defended herself with the thought that her treatment was necessary to support her therapist so that he would not die.

We are all aware of aging therapists who are themselves unaware of their failing faculties and rage at their colleagues for not referring patients to them. But one patient who was referred to such a therapist complained to the referring psychiatrist that his doctor kept falling asleep. The same is true of sick and dying therapists who are unable to separate from their patients because the patients are needed to maintain denial of their own serious illness and fear of death and separation. For these and other reasons, one woman analyst left her practice at the age of 70 and in fair health so as not to burden her patients with the possibility of her death. Another woman analyst stopped seeing psychoanalysis patients when she was 70 and shortly thereafter stopped seeing psychotherapy patients. In her late seventies and eighties, she offered her services free for supervision and teaching because she would not burden her patients with her infirmities. She died at the age of 91. However, such actions are not the norm. Retirement statistics reveal that most professionals do not think of retiring before the age of 75.

As therapists age there is usually increased physical incapacity and more loneliness. This results in the need for more object relatedness and increased dependency needs. If these needs are not met outside the treatment situation, they will be obtained within the treatment situation with disturbing consequences for the treatment process. These needs would make it more difficult for therapists to separate from their patients and terminate treatment. Such attitudes on the part of therapists will profoundly modify treatment so that it will become more supportive and less expressive. If the therapists need their patients to protect themselves from their own sense of diminished self-worth, fear of death, and increased dependency, the patients would also have great difficulty in expressing aggressive feelings for fear that someone would die. Under such circumstances it becomes difficult for patients to terminate treatment because they feel they need to support and protect the aging therapist. Such negative countertransference feelings profoundly affect the treatment process and make it imperative that the therapist be more acutely aware of his or her unmet needs, which cannot be obtained from patients because therapy will be seriously affected. Thus the need to consider retirement from teaching, training, and psychotherapy before these countertransferences develop is most essential. In addition, the use of peer consultations should be encouraged.

Summary

The effect of the psychotherapist's aging on the psychotherapeutic process may be positive or negative. Some psychotherapists become more emotionally liberated and creative, hence becoming better at their work. Others become constricted, withdrawn, dependent, angry, and depressed. Because the mind does not deteriorate as quickly as the body does, the aging psychotherapist may retain his or her skill and creativity long after physical difficulties begin.

The three cardinal principles affecting aging are health, wealth, and wisdom (or the maintenance of one's mental faculties). But the psychotherapy is markedly affected by the aura of the aging psychotherapist, and the countertransferential contaminants need to be recognized and affectively overcome in the treatment process. Grandparental transferences are different from parental ones, and patients' reactions to an aging psychotherapist need to be factored into the treatment process. As the psychotherapist becomes older there is a need to be more aware of his or her object-related needs and not to use the patient to solve such unmet needs. Consultation for a better understanding of one's countertransference difficulties should be used more often by the aging psychotherapist. I am in agreement with Eissler (1977) that the reality considerations of aging make it necessary to raise the possibility of one's death and to offer names of psychotherapists to whom patients may be referred in the event of the psychotherapist's death or a serious illness.

DEATH AND ILLNESS IN THE LIFE OF THE AGING PSYCHOTHERAPIST

Intimately connected with the aging process are the emotional reactions that develop in the psychotherapist when close relatives, especially spouses, are seriously ill and dying and how these grief reactions affect the psychotherapeutic process. In larger cities the therapist can be more anonymous. But even in cities considered large the analytic and psychotherapy community are relatively small, and critical events in the psychotherapist's life become well known to the community and the patients in therapy. Although such events can occur at any age, they usually occur more often when the psychotherapist is older.

Literature Review

As indicated earlier, discussions of these issues are only recently appearing in the literature. Several years before the publication of their article, Givelber and Simon (1981) each experienced the death of a close family member. Returning to work, they both recognized their reactions to their losses, the mourning that occurred, and the effect these feelings had on their own capacity as therapists as well as their effect on their patients. After reviewing the literature they spoke with other colleagues who had experienced similar losses. Their principal finding was that "the interaction between patient and therapist often repeats an earlier trauma for the patient in which the therapist unwittingly reenacts a pathological parental response" (p. 141). They indicated that the therapist should be sensitive to these possibilities and attempt to deal with the problem interpretively. "Rather than focusing on whether or not to reveal his or her loss to the patient, the therapist should address the broader issue of the meaning that revealing or not revealing will have for the patient" (p. 141).

Givelber and Simon (1981) also summarized several studies they found in their literature search. Balsam and Balsam (1974) emphasized that a therapist's loss may have different meanings to patients depending on the ego strength of each patient. Very ill patients are often more concerned with the absence of the therapist than with the reason behind the absence. They reported that a depressed woman was more concerned with cheering up her therapist than dealing with her problems. Rodman (1977) described the need to contain his feelings, a need that can interfere with the associations of the patient. Telling the patient something about the loss of his wife was not only necessary for him but also for his patients. However, when he communicated some of his feelings to a more seriously ill patient, the patient became so upset that the therapy was terminated. Singer (1970) chose to share some of the facts of his wife's illness and found the experience was growth promoting for his patients as they were able to show compassion for their therapist, which had not been possible earlier.

According to Givelber and Simon (1981), many therapists come back to work too soon. A large number of therapists take off no time at all. These individuals often disavow their grief reactions and find intolerable the awareness of states of their own neediness, fragility, and self-involvement. Other therapists need the structure of work to offset their loneliness and neediness, which too often involve increased object relatedness with their patients. This is similar to the description of aging therapists who, because of increased loneliness, look to their patients for fulfillment of their emotional needs. Therapists who return to work while still in active mourning are seen as fragile, sad, and depressed. This leads to an urge by the therapists to be cared for and comforted as well as an urge to more actively communicate their feelings. This in turn may result in disturbing countertransferential reactions. Such therapists may shy away from certain affects related to losses, or they may be unable to react neutrally to hostile reactions on the part of patients regarding the absences. On the other hand, there may be positive features to grief reactions on the part of therapists as well as growth-promoting features for the patient. After mourning, therapists can find psychotherapy life-affirming, which in turn increases their capacity to listen and respond to their patients' losses in a keener and more sensitive fashion.

Psychotherapists still argue about whether patients should be told of these serious events. I am convinced that telling the patient is more humane to the therapist and patient alike and beneficial to the psychotherapeutic efforts; at least there will be no need for the therapist to remain so self-contained and guard against spontaneous emotional reactions that he or she may not be able to hide.

Shapiro (1985), whose mother became ill and died, described the treatment of a male homosexual patient with problems of alcoholism. In individual therapy this patient communicated as a schizoid, fragmented, isolated person; in group therapy he was more related. At first Shapiro was involved with the serious illness of her mother and later with her grief reactions after the death. There were various transference and countertransference problems, but Shapiro never revealed the reasons for her absences or depressed moods. At times the patient saw her doze off, but he never pursued the reasons for her modified behavior. However, he talked of termination and was angry at her lack of sensitivity, but he did demonstrate grief reactions parallel to those of the therapist that were helpful in working through past traumatic losses.

These parallel mood changes in both therapist and patient continued for some time. Shapiro (1985) emphasized her increased capacity to maintain closeness with her regressed patient and resolve her own previous resistances in the psychotherapeutic process as a result of her own loss and mourning. As I read her interesting portrayal of weeks of therapy in the fifth year of treatment, I wondered whether many of the difficult periods in the therapy would have been ameliorated if the therapist had openly discussed the reasons for her mood changes and absences. The patient talked of termination, kept referring to her as mysterious, and accused her of being emotionally unavailable to support him, which was probably true.

In conclusion, Shapiro felt that the self-absorption she exhibited while coping with her loss created an atmosphere parallel to that of the patient's early life. Thus an opportunity developed for both the patient and therapist to work out their common resistances, which involved closeness and distance. I agree with Shapiro (1985) that such disturbing experiences in therapists' lives can often be used to aid their patients' work through the trauma of previous losses as these feelings are reenacted in the transference. Losses with their resultant mourning reactions can lead to liberating and growth-enhancing effects (Pollock 1981), especially as these feelings are reexperienced in therapy through the transference. The death in the life of a therapist offers a unique opportunity in the therapeutic process to work through patients' problems relating to old and traumatic losses as well as to the grief reaction of the therapist (Shapiro 1985).

Additional Data

In a personal communication, a psychoanalytic colleague described his reactions to the acute illness and death of his wife. When she was emergently taken to a hospital, he left his patients suddenly and was away from his practice for 11 days. After he returned to work for several weeks, his wife died and he was again away from his patients for about 2 weeks. Nearly all of his patients knew about the illness and death of his wife, and he was in obvious mourning. He recognized that he was irritable, more impatient, and dysphoric. But he felt more comfortable coming back to work. Looking back at that period of his life, he felt that his patients' expressions of concern helped him with his mourning reactions. In addition, he felt that he had become "softer" and more sensitive to his patients. His interpretations were less confronting and diminishing.

Another psychoanalyst, whose father had developed a cerebral vascular accident with aphasia, took 3 days off when his father died but did not tell his patients what had happened. When he returned he was surprised to hear from a candidate in training that he had checked the death notices and found out the analyst's father had died. Although the analyst originally felt he had worked out his mourning reactions when his father was ill, he was surprised that his feelings were so evident to his analysands. He said he now felt freer to tell his patients about serious incidents in his life about which grief feelings would normally develop.

Countertransference and Transference Reactions

Some years ago, my wife was diagnosed as having a life-threatening form of cancer. The early treatment program included two abdominal operations and months of chemotherapy, resulting in my having many weekly periods away from my practice. Because the majority of my patients were aware of the illness, there was no option as to whether I should or should not tell them what had happened. Despite my obvious grief reactions, I did not respond to questions about my own feelings, nor did I offer any information about the subsequent course of my wife's illness. However, during the continuing intensive treatment procedures, my wife's serious physical changes were noted and reacted to by my patients.

The early obvious effect of my wife's illness on me was noted by my friends, relatives, and patients. I was seen as ill, aged, unempathic, and not listening, which frequently was true. I was accused of forgetfulness, which was also true, and I made errors in my interpretations because my capacity for listening and being sensitive to the usual clues in therapy had temporarily disappeared. I recognized my increased irritability, especially to those patients who were acting out, who were in a negative phase of treatment, or who were so ill that they made little reference to my wife's illness but were angered at my absences. Some of my interpretations to these patients were hostile and diminishing and I felt burnt out by my patients' problems. I began to seriously think of retirement as a response to my grief reactions and the "burdens of my patients."

The initial reaction by most of my patients was grave concern for my wife and my reactions to her illness. These feelings were frequently followed by fears of separation and the possibility of the termination of therapy, especially by those patients who had suffered earlier traumatic separations and losses. They felt I would be leaving my practice to take care of my wife. Nearly all of the patients with better ego strengths felt their symptoms and complaints were trivial compared with my real problems: "How can I talk about my insignificant problems if you are so burdened?" There was considerable resistance to free association and the uncovering of other conflicts in patients, and there was marked resistance to the development of further transferential material.

The following case examples illustrate patients' transference reactions to my wife's illness and my countertransference behavior. Most patients were aware of my wife's illness, but there were a few who were unaware of the situation or were so ill or narcissistic that they were not aware of my change in mood.

Case 1

Ms. A and Ms. B (see Case 2 below), two patients who were close to termination, made it clear to me that they would not leave me when I needed so much support. After all, I had supported them when they needed my help. Both women knew each other and had talked about the situation. They also both came from dysfunctional families and suffered disturbing earlier separations and losses.

Ms. A, who had previously been in analysis, but was now in once-a-week psychotherapy, suffered an absence from her father during World War II for more than 3 years. When he returned he seemed disinterested in her, but a sister was born who became the father's pet and the favorite in the family. Ms. A's mother was constantly critical and diminished anything she did; her father was passive and unavailable. Ms. A, who was very attractive, developed anxiety reactions, phobias, and a poor sense of self with narcissistic symptoms, depreciating all her qualities except her physical attractiveness. During the earlier years of treatment, both her parents died of cancer, and there was some resolution of her earlier rivalrous relationship with her sister, who saw Ms. A as a mother substitute.

During the middle period of my wife's illness, Ms. A had the following dream: "I was sitting next to you at the opera. You were alone and told me you had two tuxedos made and discussed the one you were wearing. I thought how odd, you and I were talking and reacting to one another like two close friends. Then I found myself intensely crying because your wife was ill. I cared so much for you because of your suffering. Then I felt you were right in telling me that I was suffering from sibling rivalry. I was beating up on W. [a substitute for her sister but a daughter of her male friend]. She said, 'Dad is going into therapy to understand you.' I said, 'He is going into therapy for you, not me,' and I laid into her again."

Ms. A's associations had to do with her close warm feelings toward me, aroused by the threat of an offer for a good position in another city where she would be separated from me. She associated to an incident in her teens in which she had slapped her sister for taking her television seat. She recognized her overreaction to her sister as being related to her anger toward her father, for not being available to her, and her anger toward me, for threatening to separate from her because of my wife, a more successful rival. She could not accept the new offer away from home and therapy, but my grief reaction facilitated her in dealing with earlier traumas related to her losses and separations, as well as her intense sibling rivalry, especially as it related to W.

Case 2

At first, Ms. B, who was in the terminating phase of a long analysis, refused to consider leaving treatment because of my need for support during my wife's illness. However, her earlier, more severe reactions to separations began to surface and affect her. Much analytic work related to her previous losses and separation, and the projected separation from me was emotionally reacted to and interpreted in the transference. It seemed evident that the serious illness in my life was a significant catalyst to further work in analysis as regarded her concerns about losses and separation. Termination occurred despite the continued illness of my wife.

Case 3

Ms. C, who was in her late fifties and had been in analysis for 3 years, was particularly upset by my wife's illness and early on would obtain information about my wife from common friends to keep in touch with the progress of her treatment. When she originally came for analysis, she spoke of her lifelong feelings of diminished self-worth, dysphoric feelings, and overcritical attitudes toward her friends and her husband. She had been in psychotherapy off and on for many years before coming to see me. Her mother was also overcritical, felt depreciated, and was compulsive in her behavior. Her father felt diminished, overdrank, and was passive and emotionally unavailable for close and affectionate interactions with his daughter. Although Ms. C was attractive as a youngster, she always felt drab and unattractive, especially as compared with her younger brother who was the "golden boy" at home and in the community. Closeness and intimacy were always problems with her friends and in therapy as well.

In the early phase of my wife's illness, Ms. C was in great emotional turmoil. During treatment both her father and mother died, and she had the entire burden of both illnesses because her brother lived out of town and was emotionally uninvolved with his dying parents. Also, before treatment began, Ms. C had had breast cancer and a breast was removed.

Ms. C developed competitive feelings with anyone who had information she did not have about my wife. One day she became angry when another of my patients called me by my first name, as she could not allow herself to do. She also felt diminished by me as she felt I was more involved with the other patient, perhaps giving information she was being refused. Showing any kind of feeling to me was most difficult for her, but this increased after my wife became ill because she was even more frightened that showing angry feelings toward me would cause my wife to die. This was similar to how she reacted as a child: always conforming, never showing anger, and anxious to please her family so nothing frightening would happen at home. That was why she constantly needed to know the state of my wife's health.

We finally agreed that she would refrain from seeking information about my wife and face her anxiety. Shortly after this agreement, Ms. C broke out in anger: "Why does your wife have to be so sick and take you away from me?" She finally could admit that she was worried about losing me and very jealous of my attention to my wife. We talked about the strain of her mother's death and her own fears of cancer. Then she wondered about her anger. She recognized that she felt guilty about her warm and intimate feelings for me, and the thought had occurred to her that if my wife died I would be available to her as a love object. Working through these transference reactions resulted in an increased ability for Ms. C to show warmth, as well as healthy anger toward me, her husband, and her friends. The serious illness of my wife allowed for an arousal of her repressed anger and for warm and intimate feelings to emerge, reducing her critical behavior and enabling her to accept herself and the people around her as they were, instead of how she perceived that she or others ought to be.

Some time after my wife's illness, we began to talk about termination. Ms. C had some regression and return of her symptoms, asking questions about my wife's illness again, although there had been no ongoing treatment for some time. We talked of her difficulty in separating from me.

Shortly thereafter Ms. C saw a photograph exhibit that included a picture depicting cancer; part of the picture was a naked woman and a hospital. Ms. C was intensely moved to tears after viewing this picture and grieved not only for my wife but her own disfigured body. Associating to her intense emotional reaction to the picture, she was reminded of the fact that she was angry with her husband and again speculated that if my wife died she could divorce her husband and marry me. All of these thoughts and feelings had become more intense since we talked of termination. Ms. C wondered how I could cope with the thought of separating from my wife. We continued discussing her fear of termination and separation from me. I suggested that the possible loss of my wife was raising concerns in her as to whether I had any feelings about separating from her, as she was so upset and depressed about leaving me. We spoke of the inevitability of losses and separations.

With an increased sense of self as a result of her developing insight and new identification, Ms. C began to report increased gratifications in her life. She was able to bring up happy memories of her parents and even her brother who had recently returned to live with his wife and was thus less available as a close friend. Relatives were always very important to her because she had no children and only two or three cousins.

Ms. C's repetitive reenactments in the transference of her reactions to loss, stimulated by the illness of my wife, helped to slowly repair her damaged sense of self and increase her feeling of autonomy. Her old panic concerning my wife lessened, and she became more comfortable with closeness, her inner feelings, and an increased sense of self. Moreover, during this period of the analysis, although my wife was still ill, I was able to enjoy life with less pain and was more available for sensitive listening, more empathic, less irritable, and more able to accommodate to my own potential loss and separation.

Case 4

Mr. D, a patient in his late forties, had an earlier diagnosis of schizophrenia and exhibited symptoms of a borderline personality disorder. His reactions to my wife's illness as well as to those of his close relatives were without much conscious feeling. Although occasionally apologizing for his lack of concern about my wife, his feelings regarding my absences were more correlated to his own fear of losing a selfobject so important to his survival that he could not identify with my distress. His need to overcome his inner feelings of being ugly, physically deformed (untrue), and without social presence was so strong that he had no capacity to use the fact of my wife's illness as an enactment of his past serious traumas.

Summary

Although psychotherapists vary in their reactions to death in their lives, nearly all exhibit the symptoms of mourning. It would be wiser if mourning psychotherapists stayed away from their practice until they became stable enough emotionally that inappropriate emotional reactions in the psychotherapeutic situation would be less likely to occur. Containing emotional reactions without letting patients know what has happened produces more countertransference reactions and will affect psychotherapy adversely. Most patients are aware, consciously or unconsciously, that their therapist is mourning, and lack of information prevents the resolution of problems that arise in therapy.

When a psychotherapist denies such significant episodes in his or her life, the patient avoids them also, and the psychotherapeutic situation becomes burdened by the lack of the patient's information about the changed emotional attitudes of the therapist. The patient's expression of feelings and free associations will give way to the need to support the therapist with the avoidance of facing conflicts within and without the patient. The patient's symptoms may become trivialized in the face of the psychotherapist's grief reactions. With more open communications, more affect-laden feelings can be better reacted to by patient and therapist alike. The patient's reactions to death in the psychotherapist's life will vary with the intensity of the psychopathology in the patient. Effectively working through the therapist's grief and mourning reactions in the process of psychotherapy may lead to an enhancement of the empathy and sensitivity of the therapist and may be helpful in working through significant losses and separations in the patient (Pollock 1981).

THE DYING PSYCHOTHERAPIST

Although the psychotherapist, like everyone, is subject to life-threatening illness that do lead to death, almost no articles have been published that deal with the experiences of the terminal phase of an illness and their effect on the therapeutic process. We have all heard vignettes by observers of dying psychotherapists who deny the existence of the serious illness and continue to see their patients even when they are close to death. Freud stopped seeing patients only several weeks before his death (Lord et al. 1978). An analyst with a cancer of the head of his pancreas, who lost weight and became jaundiced, denied the concerns of his patients, said he had hepatitis, and died without preparing his patients for his serious illness or transfer to a colleague. Another, who looked so drugged at a conference that his friends queried him about his health, said it was excellent. He later set up analytic time with patients for the fall but died during the summer. I mentioned above two women analysts who retired after age 70 so as not to burden their analysands with their illnesses and death, which were not in evidence at that time. It seems to me that these individuals are in the minority. Few psychotherapists seek consultation about problems concerning their aging, about their responses to death in their lives, or when they are suffering serious life-threatening illnesses.

Literature Review

Why have analysts and psychotherapists commonly avoided discussing such an important issue, one that develops so frequently in the psychotherapeutic process? In their bibliographic review, Lord et al. (1978) noted that Freud had emphasized that one cannot conceive of his or her own death and that physicians particularly are loath to come to terms with the actuality of death because they are dedicated to the prevention of it. In addition, they noted that Eissler had spoken of a physician's death as "something negative, a deficit, the absence of something" (p. 149). Burton (1967) described a study in which 300 psychoanalysts selected at random were asked about their attitudes toward death. The brevity of their remarks and some of the anger expressed in the responses suggested marked resistance to the topic. The lack of any discussion of this topic in medical schools is also a factor. Halpert (1982) emphasized some of the defenses that come into play when a therapist is fatally ill, such as isolation and denial because of their narcissistic mortifications of having to face separation. Halpert also felt that even Freud is used as a role model because he was sick for years but maintained his practice without facing the countertransference aspects of his serious illness on his patients.

Lord et al. (1978) used questionnaires to survey 27 analysands whose analysts had died in the midst of their treatment. Their subsequent analysts were also contacted by questionnaires. The authors found that reactions to sudden death were more pronounced and that older analysands, longer in treatment with past histories of significant losses and separations, reacted more severely. Ten analysands developed severe grief reactions (symptoms of mourning for more than a year). Eleven analysands had a normal mourning reaction. Noncandidate analysands suffered severe mourning reactions twice as often as candidate analysands. The younger analysands who were in the early stages of their analyses suffered fewer reactions. Those analysands who had some knowledge of their analysts' illness before the death also had fewer reactions. Their findings "affirm the concept that the analysand's mourning process does not derive solely from the broken and unresolved transferred relations to the psychoanalyst. It is also significantly based on the loss of the analyst experienced as a human being in his own right" (Lord et al. 1978, p. 195).

Halpert (1982) reported on two patients who were seen by him and another analyst after their previous analysts had died or suspended treatment because of a terminal illness. Both previous analysts did not reveal the seriousness of their illnesses. Halpert described the countertransference aspects present in the dying psychoanalyst who used denial, isolation, and narcissistic withdrawal as defenses, so that the analyst's neutrality, objectivity, and empathy were substantially impaired. He quoted Eissler as stating that "when the analyst denies his own illness it seems inevitable that the patient denies it too" (Halpert 1982, p. 388).

Eissler (1977) emphasized the need for the aging or dying psychoanalyst to plan for death by giving his analysands referral sources. Although a patient's concern about the possibility of the death of the therapist may be related to psychopathology, reality factors must also be dealt with without countertransference behavior on the part of the therapist. Few therapists plan for their own deaths. There has been much discussion about the pros and cons of disclosure to patients about nonfatal illnesses of the therapist (see Chapter 2), but Halpert (1982) emphasized the need for disclosure if the therapist is dying so that the inevitability of a final separation can be worked through in the therapeutic process.

Clinical Research Study

In July 1980, Dr. David Rothman—an obstetrician and gynecologist who had considerable training in psychotherapy and saw patients in psychotherapy every afternoon—developed a malignant lymphoma of one of his kidneys. Following 6 weeks of radiation therapy, he was supposed to receive chemotherapy, but he had to postpone that treatment because of a low white blood cell count. Late in October 1980, a metastases to his neck was removed, and in December 1980, after 2 months of chemotherapy, all of his hair fell out. In a paper, written in the spring of 1981, he described the therapeutic use of his terminal illness to help his patients work through their earlier losses and separations by working through the inevitable separation from him. In the summer of 1981, he asked me to read and critique his paper. I made several suggestions, mainly related to the need for more past history and a better description of his patients' earlier therapeutic experiences.

Unfortunately, he was too seriously ill to accomplish this task, and he died 28 February 1982.

I had no further thoughts about his paper until early in 1983. Obviously my mourning for the death of my close friend interfered with my ability to show any active interest as to what happened to the paper. But with my renewed capacity for work after the mourning process, I obtained the unpublished manuscript and asked for permission to look through his records. This was difficult because his records were unnamed for reasons of confidentiality. I finally found the five patients he had discussed and discovered that he had kept notes on all his patients, even for some of them during the month preceding his death. It became clear to me that he had not separated from his patients before his death, long after the cutoff date in his paper (the spring of 1981). After the summer of 1981, there were many canceled appointments, some unannounced, but neither the therapist nor his patients could successfully arrange for a planned termination of treatment. However, during this difficult period, Rothman continued to keep ongoing notes of his treatment hours. During the years of his psychotherapeutic experience, he had had regular supervision from one or more psychoanalysts.

Recognizing Rothman's serious countertransferences that had prevented a planned separation from taking place, I decided to conduct an intensive study of his thesis and his clinical notes and to try to obtain interviews with the five patients he used in his study. During interviews of the five patients, I discovered that three of them had seen other therapists (from whom I obtained information as well). Previous articles relating to the topic of the dying psychotherapist had used questionnaires or information from subsequent therapists, but none had used the therapist's original notes and interviews with the patients to understand the psychotherapeutic process.

Rothman indicated in his paper that all his patients, four of whom were seen twice a week, knew that he had cancer. He had been out of the office 3 weeks after the original surgery. Although his patients' reaction to his surgery was one of concern, he felt it was only after the loss of his hair that intense reactions began to appear: "This was most marked in three patients who had periods of depression that were severe enough to cause withdrawal from their usual activities, fortunately for a short period of time. In the other two women, there was anxiety over the threat of separation but with a less intense reaction. One difference noted in these two groups is that in the three patients with marked reactive depression, there had been more severe early losses and deprivations, with rejection by both parents, whereas, in the other two patients there had been a more supportive relationship with at least one parent" (Kaplan and Rothman 1986, p. 563).

Communication of the terminal illness.   Although all of Rothman's patients were in some way aware of his terminal illness, they were unanimous in their reactions that he had never used the word *cancer* and that his denial of the severity of the illness made it impossible for them to admit the facts to themselves. However, Rothman felt he had communicated his severe illness to his patients in a straightforward way. His optimism caused them to deny the reality of the situation: "What seemed clear from this study is that the communication of the terminal illness will be defended against by both the patients and their psychotherapist unless a planned termination of treatment before the therapist's forced incapacity is undertaken. This will allow for a re-emergence and working through of the repressed grief, anger, and hopelessness and other fantasies that accompany mourning and will also facilitate referral to another psychotherapist, ideally while the first therapist is still alive" (Kaplan and Rothman 1986, p. 570).

Grief reactions.   Two of the patients, who were older, had more depressive symptoms, and had suffered more earlier losses and separations, developed prolonged grief reactions after Rothman's death. These were patients who had been in treatment longer and had known their therapist longer: "The study corroborates the results of Lord et al. (1978) who found that older patients, those longer in treatment, and those who had suffered more severe early deprivation were more likely to develop more severe grief reactions, sometimes leading to prolonged mourning. However, the study also indicates that another important variable seems to be the severity of the depressive symptoms present at the time of referral which also coincides with the intensity of the grief reactions" (Kaplan and Rothman 1986, p. 570).

Use of the terminal illness as a therapeutic tool.   It is a tribute to Rothman's courage that he was able to use his terminal illness to help his patients with their past losses and separation. Despite the difficulty in accepting the reality of their therapist's death, four of the five patients felt that they had been able for the first time to work through the repressed and unworked-out emotional reactions to the earlier deaths of and separation or abandonment from their caretakers. But one patient said that "a more significant catharsis would have been possible if [Rothman] had been able to allow me to grieve for him in a more personal way"; this would have allowed her to interact with him more realistically, which "would have been significant for me and, I think, also for him" (Kaplan and Rothman 1986, p. 570). The patients were angry that they were not able to mourn their loving and respected therapist while he was alive. Rothman's continued use of the mourning reaction to help his patients was also a defense to deny his own need to face the reality of his death and inevitable separation.

Transference and countertransference reactions.   Rothman had reported in his paper on his earlier inability to accept the reality of his own deteriorating illness. In one case report he described his helplessness, his depression, and the anger his illness had produced and how his attitudes affected his communication with his patients. In response to one patient who was fearful that he would not be at the office when she arrived, he "felt like yelling, 'But I am not dying. I am hoping for a cure. Don't dispose of me so quickly'" (Kaplan and Rothman 1986, p. 570).

Rothman's inability to arrange for a planned separation (a forced termination) is indicative of his countertransference feelings of denial, isolation, and narcissistic withdrawal that made it difficult for his patients to face separation. He needed his patients to reassure himself about his own viability as much as they needed him to be alive and well. As a result he became increasingly unaware of the burden his deteriorating condition had on his patients. They, however, were acutely aware of this burden but avoided separation out of the need to care for their therapist as a beloved parent. One patient, feeling intense anger, helplessness, and dysphoria coupled with denial and compulsive behavior, began to fear the death of her close relatives. In her fantasies she saw herself as Rothman's favorite child. She had a dream in which she was Anna Freud (then alive), the favorite child closely involved with her father, Sigmund Freud.

Other patients reacted to the impending death in idiosyncratic ways related to their personality and psychopathology. Besides grief, one patient developed increased sexual and masochistic fantasies to encourage a closer and continuous relationship with her therapist to avoid separation. On the other hand, she guiltily wished for his death so she could mourn without ambivalence. Inappropriate acting-out behavior was followed by increased sexual feelings. Another patient felt angry and abused, like a child who had suffered physical abuse. She had moderate dysphoric symptoms. She also dreamt of her children dying and had a severe reaction to the death of a friend, which was accentuated because of her feelings about her therapist. One of the five patients had no mourning reaction. She had become pregnant and delivered a child during her treatment, which she felt was "elective." No significant transference had developed and the treatment was shorter. When she read of Rothman's death in the newspaper, she was somewhat upset but "not for herself but for Rothman's courageous behavior in carrying out psychotherapy while terminally ill" (Kaplan and Rothman 1986, p. 571).

The two therapists who saw three of the patients after Rothman died felt that not enough attention had been paid to the real situation. They described two of their patients as being in prolonged mourning. One of the patients became pregnant shortly after seeing her new therapist and terminated therapy. She told me that she could not develop a significant alliance with the new therapist and that the coming of the new baby made the therapy seem insignificant. One patient in subsequent therapy remarked that "it would have been better if [Rothman] had been able to accept the reality of the situation, but I recognize that would have been asking too much" (Kaplan and Rothman 1986, p. 571).

SUMMARY

When a therapist is terminally ill, grief reactions will develop in the patient and therapist alike. The severity of the grief reactions in patients will depend on the length of time in treatment, the age of the patient, the extent of earlier deprivations, and the intensity of depressive symptoms present at the time of referral. Terminal illness takes a toll on the therapist and patient. The burden of the physical and mental changes in the therapist makes it impossible for patients to bring up issues that must seem trivial and to show anger to their therapist. At the same time, the therapist's capacity for neutrality, empathy, introspection, access to his or her own affects, and sensitivity to the patients' associations are all severely limited. Unless a planned termination of treatment takes place, the communication of a terminal illness becomes obscure, and neither therapist nor patient can accept the reality of the situation.

Eissler (1977) suggested that the aging psychoanalyst who cannot perform his or her normal activities should inform the patient of the reality. Then, after several weeks in which the patient's fantasies and feelings are explored, the patient should be referred to another therapist. According to Eissler this should be done before too much deterioration has occurred, so the patient could be in the second therapy while the first therapist is alive (see Halpert 1982). This is certainly true for the dying psychotherapist. This would give the patient an opportunity to mourn the first therapist during the forced termination but would facilitate the working through of the grief reactions with the second therapist. It might even be possible for the patient to be discharged by the first therapist. Obviously "all of these comments rest on the assumption that the therapist's own countertransference and physical condition do not preclude an ability to face his or her own serious illness" (Kaplan and Rothman 1986, pp. 571–572).

References

Balsam RM, Balsam A: Becoming a Psychotherapist: A Clinical Primer, Boston, MA, Little, Brown, 1974

Birren JE: A contribution to the psychology of aging: as a counterpart of development, in Emergent Theories of Aging. Edited by Birren JE, Berngtson VL. New York, Springer Publishing, 1988, pp 153–176

Burton A: Death as a countertransference. Psychoanalysis and the Psychoanalytic Review 49(4):3–20, 1962

Eissler KR: On the possible effects of aging on the practice of psychoanalysis: an essay. Journal of the Philadelphia Association for Psychoanalysis 3:138–152, 1977

Givelber F, Simon B: Death in the life of a psychotherapist. Psychiatry 44:141–149, 1981

Halpert E: When the analyst is chronically ill or dying. Psychoanal Q 51:372–389, 1982

Kaplan AH, Rothman D: The dying psychotherapist. Am J Psychiatry 143:561–572, 1986

Lord R, Ritvo S, Solnit AZ: Patients' reactions to the death of the psychoanalyst. Int J Psychoanal 59:189–197, 1978

Pollock GH: Aging or aged, in The Course of Life: Adulthood and the Aging Process, Vol 3. Edited by Greenspan SI, Pollock GH. Washington, DC, U.S. Department of Health and Human Services, 1981, pp 549–585

Rodman FR: Not Dying. New York, Random House, 1977

Shapiro R: A case study: the terminal illness and death of the analyst's mother: its effect on her treatment of a severely regressed patient. Modern Psychoanalysis 10:31–45, 1985

Singer E: The patients aids the analyst: some clinical and theoretical observations, in The Name of Life: Essays in Honor of Erich Fromm. Edited by Landis B, Tauber E. Fort Worth, TX, Holt, Rinehart and Winston, 1970

Chapter 4

The Therapist's Absences

Carol C. Nadelson, M.D.

Psychotherapists are absent from their practices for a variety of reasons, including illness and vacations, as well as personal and professional obligations and responsibilities. There has been much informal speculation about the impact of absences on patients; however, there is a very sparse literature on this subject, consisting primarily of anecdotal material and clinical reports. This literature focuses primarily on absences related to therapist illness or life events like pregnancy or on therapists' leaving because of geographic relocation (Abend 1982; Dahlberg 1980; Eissler 1977; Givelber and Simon 1981; Hannett 1949; Kriechman 1984; Nadelson et al. 1974). There are no published articles related to absence because of professional obligations.

REASONS FOR THERAPIST ABSENCES

It is important to consider the reasons for absences because the issues raised appear to differ in different situations. When the reason for an absence is a life event (e.g., illness), it is generally viewed as out of the control of the therapist or analyst. Expectable life-phase events (e.g., pregnancy or graduations) are also seen as not under direct control. Professional obligations or moving a location of practice are events that can be attributed to the personal needs, narcissism, ambition, or nontherapeutic interests of the therapist. Because such reasons often support career advances or provide external rewards or recognition, they are often considered to be countertherapeutic for the patient, despite the lack of evidence to support this position. In addition, because absences can stimulate a range of ambivalent feelings in colleagues and patients, including envy, competitiveness, and even anger, it is not surprising that this view is held and often reinforces the guilt of the therapist.

71

Another group of frequent (in fact almost routine) absences that are rarely written about or discussed are those attributed to institutional or training requirements. They are also seen as out of the therapist's control and include transfers and terminations that occur during training, when residents leave a program or change rotations, or when staff are assigned to other services. Keith (1966) wrote about the "transfer syndrome," which he suggested is common in clinical parlance but neglected in standard textbooks of psychotherapy. He speculated that this neglect occurs because the authors of such texts tend to practice long-term psychotherapy or psychoanalysis and do not transfer patients very often. Pumpian-Mindlin (1958) suggested that therapists' need for success may result in setting unrealistic therapeutic goals for patients and blaming administrative authorities for interruptions in treatment. A solution to the problems caused by multiple transfers of patients, according to Reider (1953), is to encourage patients to develop positive transference feelings to an institution instead of, or in addition to those, to an individual.

THERAPEUTIC NEUTRALITY AND PERSONAL DISCLOSURE

Among the important theoretical considerations in therapy is the concept of therapeutic neutrality. Over the past few decades, our thinking about therapeutic neutrality has been modified (although not abandoned), recognizing that in more absolute terms, it is unrealistic. After all, the choice of our office location, its decor, our dress and manner, and the way in which we run our practices are open to the patient. Each creates an impression and has meaning to the patient. We have all experienced a patient who criticized our choice of art, the way we do our billing, or even our manner on the telephone. Likewise, despite our efforts, we can never avoid being a public presence. A chance encounter at the same supermarket, a PTA meeting, or professional seminar is inevitable. As our presence affects our patients, so does our absence. Thus therapeutic neutrality relates more to direct disclosure of personal information than to other means of learning about the therapist.

In discussing what he called "special events" in therapy (e.g., encounters in nonoffice settings), Weiss (1975) indicated that in some way these events all intrude on the therapeutic process. He noted that many special events are so common and routine that they are forgotten. He emphasized, however, that they do have a therapeutic impact. Psychoanalytic candidates, for example, who see their analysts in seminars and conferences, are affected by the transference issues. Mishandling these encounters in therapy or analysis, Weiss suggested, may damage the therapeutic interaction. He noted that "when 'special events' take place many patients appear to remain oblivious and silent to the intrapsychic clash between the analyst as a real figure and the analyst as a transference object" (p. 75).

Apart from planned vacations or an occasional illness, many therapists first come to encounter the impact of their absence through a life event like a pregnancy, an illness, or a family crisis. Most therapists find individual solutions in their work with patients. They are concerned about what and how to tell their patients. When there is a pregnancy or an injury, part of the question is addressed by its visibility. But, what if one is preoccupied, erratic in attention or presence, or unable to keep previous commitments because of a life tragedy?

In discussing disclosure to a patient, Weiner (1972) indicated that self-exposure should be tied to the specific need of the patient at a given moment and this must be made clear in the therapy. Gitleson (1952) noted that an impasse in an analysis can occur because the analyst does not recognize, misunderstands, or avoids the patient's perception of him or her as a real person.

In revealing facts about his marriage, Flaherty (1979) suggested that patients would discover the fact themselves if not told, and he considered failure to reveal the facts to be a breach of the alliance. He believed that with sicker patients there may be more of a need to allow the patient to discover the therapist as a real person and for the patient to tolerate the feelings he or she may have about the therapist.

IMPACT OF THERAPEUTIC ABSENCE

Chernin (1976) suggested that with planned absences the therapist maintains control but that interruptions of therapy secondary to illness find both patient and therapist unprepared, and the therapist often feels that he or she has lost control. In discussing termination precipitated by a geographic move, Dewald (1965, 1966) indicated that it can represent an arbitrary decision by the analyst based on his or her personal interests and needs and does not take into account the potential impact on the patient or whether the patient has clinical indications for termination. If an event comes suddenly and unexpectedly, the reality of the analyst's life is introduced, and the event can become a stressful and traumatic reality. It may repeat infantile and childhood helplessness in the face of arbitrary parental behavior and feelings of rejection and desertion. Because the analyst had urged patients to trust and emotionally invest in him or her, with the implied promise that the analysis would continue to the point of an appropriate conclusion, the trust is broken by the termination.

Dewald (1965, 1966, 1982) further suggested that there is a difference between patients in supportive therapy, who verbalize positive transference feelings as well as sadness, regret, and concern, and those in insight-oriented therapy, who may have more negative reactions, including rage and anger about desertion and abandonment. He emphasized that unless countertransference issues are recognized and dealt with, the therapist may find it difficult to help the patient deal effectively with reactions. Both therapist and patient can conspire to avoid recognition or verbalization of reactions to the event. The most significant factor may be the therapist's guilt about deserting the patient.

Rosenbaum (1977) studied a group of psychoanalysts who moved to distant cities. Although they attempted to transfer their patients to colleagues, most patients refused. The analysts continued their contact with the patients by phone and correspondence. He suggested that certain patients cannot mourn fully and therefore cannot relinquish the therapist, remaining dependent and attached. This, he believed, was not in any way related to a particular diagnostic category.

A STUDY

To better understand the issues involving voluntary absences of therapists, I chose to approach my colleagues' experiences by asking them to respond to some questions about it. Their interest in engaging on the topic was reflected in their enthusiastic responses.

I constructed a brief questionnaire and sent it to colleagues around the United States and Canada who I knew were absent from their psychotherapy or psychoanalytic practices for a myriad of professional reasons. In some cases I conducted a personal interview in addition to or instead of the questionnaire. My purpose was to ascertain whether there were prevailing points of view, common concerns, or patterns or observations that would contribute to our understanding of this subject. I was also interested in the particular patient characteristics, if any, that could be identified as problematic, or the situations that therapists identified as more troublesome. I did not use a random sample for data collection, nor do my efforts represent a scientific study; however, perhaps these impressions will initiate a more systematic inquiry into the subject.

A group of 30 colleagues ranging in age from 40 to 80 years and including 15 male and 15 female psychotherapists and psychoanalysts

(M.D.s and Ph.D.s) were included in my sample. All of those I contacted continued active clinical practice despite absences from their offices ranging from days to months in addition to their regular vacation periods of 2–4 weeks a year. Most respondents indicated that they were intermittently away for professional meetings, for no longer than a few days at a time, but several times a year. Several had taken sabbaticals of several months.

There was wide geographic diversity represented, and most of the subjects lived in urban areas. The group was equally divided between those who practiced both long-term psychotherapy and psychoanalysis and those who did not have psychoanalytic training and were primarily psychotherapists. More than 80% of the sample had had personal psychotherapy or psychoanalysis. There was no difference in response related to whether they were or were not psychoanalysts.

To improve the response rate and the substance of responses I limited the number and type of questions I asked. In addition to collecting demographic data and other specific information about practice and personal history, the questionnaire contained brief essay questions, which I summarize below.

"Have You Shared the Reasons for Absences With Your Patients? What Do You See as the Pros and Cons of Doing So?"

Only 2 of the 30 subjects stated that they do not tell their patients the reasons for their absences, and only 1 of these responded with a categorical no. There were a diversity of responses and many qualifications, but the respondents generally focused on whether the patients specifically asked about the nature of the absence. In the context of therapy, the reasons for asking were explored with the patients and answers were given. Almost all stated that they did not provide elaborate detail or expand beyond what they judged to be accurate and sufficient. Most commented that lying or evasion seemed far more damaging to the therapeutic relationship than being truthful. Many stated that earlier in their careers they felt that disclosure was not a good idea, but over time they had changed their views and now felt that it was both fair and helpful in their treatment of patients. Several of the respondents indicated that most of their patients entered therapy knowing in advance that this pattern was to be expected.

These responses suggest that current practice may differ from traditional theoretical models of psychodynamic psychotherapy in which regular and more or less uninterrupted periods of time have been considered to be essential to the process. Changes in therapeutic practice and the use of short-term psychotherapies have generated questions, particularly about outcomes related to continuity and interruptions in therapy. It has also been suggested that patients who are new to therapy may see the pattern they negotiate as the appropriate and even the best way to engage in therapy.

The following case example illustrates a patient's confrontation with an issue that had not been addressed previously, precipitated by her therapist's absence:

Case 1

Ms. A, a 32-year-old lawyer, entered therapy with concerns about her 8-year relationship with a man she had met in law school. She felt that the relationship had soured, but she could not end it because she was unable to make any change in her life that necessitated leaving a place or a person to whom she had become attached. In fact, she lived down the street from her parents, where she had grown up. She had attended college and law school in the same city, and although she had made new friends, she continued many of her early relationships despite a lack of compatibility or interest. She felt burdened by her inability to make changes and wanted help.

From the beginning of the therapy, Ms. A was informed by the therapist that there would be absences related to professional obligations. Initially, she was relieved because she often made short business trips, and it seemed reasonable to her to negotiate definite times for meetings around both schedules. Despite this plan, though, Ms. A became increasingly anxious each time the therapist was absent.

In the course of the therapy, Ms. A revealed that from early in her childhood her parents traveled frequently and left her with a grandmother. They were very close until her grandmother died suddenly, in her presence, when she was 10 years old. At that time, she began to suffer severe anxiety symptoms when any separation occurred, and she started treatment. She did well for a 2-year period, in a very regular psychotherapeutic relationship. After the therapy was terminated, she continued to see the therapist informally because he lived in her neighborhood. She avoided relationships that might involve separating from her family and environment.

In her current therapy she recalled that she felt that she had never confronted separation in her adult life, until the current therapeutic situation, when her therapist briefly left for an out-of-town meeting. The therapy focused on these issues in the context of periodic separations and ultimately enabled the patient to deal with this aspect of her life so that she could make choices about relationships.

Another important issue that emerged from the study was the impact of the length of the therapist's absence, although times were not specifically stated.[1] One respondent indicated that patients should be told specific details of longer absences because "long absences can arouse substantial, and not so useful, anxiety levels when patients don't know whether you are sick, how sick, etc., or on vacation. Whereas with short absences there is less need for such involvement with your personal life and the fantasies and feelings are productively explorable."

Many of the respondents discussed the meaning of disclosure to patients. Several suggested that the patient might be unduly burdened by disclosure and wondered if it was, at times, the therapist's ambivalence or guilt that provoked it, rather than concern about the patient's response to separation, as is often the stated consideration. One respondent noted that if absences are an integral part of a career, it is not in the patient's interest for the therapist to be apologetic, guilty, or defensive or to see absences as calamitous.

Most of the therapists who took small trips related to their professional responsibilities stated that they tried, whenever possible, to reschedule their patients. Several indicated that because they changed appointments, they were also more flexible with patients and rescheduled and accepted changes their patients requested. Many of these therapists reported seeing patients who also traveled because of their work.

Most of us are aware that traditional models for psychodynamic psychotherapy generally fail to take account of irregular work and travel schedules that are part of the lives of many patients as well as of many therapists. It may be that some patients are dissuaded from entering therapy because their past experience has been that therapists are inflexible. As the following case example illustrates, a good therapeutic alliance coupled with discussion of issues to be thought about during the absence can be productive and enable the therapist and patient to pick up where they left off:

Case 2

Mr. B, a 42-year-old executive employed by a multinational corporation, began therapy when he became seriously depressed for the first time in his life. He had always been active and had moved frequently to different parts of the world. He had recently married and his depression appeared to have been precipitated by "settling down." Mr. B was started on an antidepressant and was seen weekly for a 2-month period. He improved dramatically over this time. He wanted to pursue psychotherapy, how-

---

[1] The delineations "long" or "brief" were not specific, but most respondents appeared to define long absences as longer than usual vacations. Frequent absences appeared to mean being absent for a session every few weeks.

ever, because he feared that he might have a recurrence if he did not have a better understanding of the reasons for his depression. Regular sessions began and he was gradually tapered off antidepressants.

About a month later Mr. B went on a business trip that would last 6 weeks. He was eager to use some of his time to think about himself. When he returned he produced a journal, stating that the regular entries had been productive and organizing for him. Over the course of the next 2 years of therapy he was gone several additional times, as was his therapist. On each reencounter it was possible to pick up and continue the therapeutic work.

Many therapists also reported that they attempted to be available to their patients in the event of an emergency or crisis, even when they were away. Some had call-in times that were formally adhered to; others were called only in an emergency. Some indicated that they kept in touch with patients by sending postcards, although one respondent questioned whether this fostered dependency.

"Have You Seen Positive and/or Negative Effects of Your Absences on Patients? Can You Be Specific About Circumstances and Types of Reactions? Are There Differences in Patients' Responses Based on Age, Gender, Diagnosis, or Other Factors?"

Most of the respondents felt that the effects of absences were both positive and negative, but there were very few who reported serious negative consequences. They almost universally concluded that they had anticipated more difficulty than they found. Some reported advantages, including the mobilization of affect, such as anger, that often enabled patients to deal with issues of separation, dependency, and omnipotence. Many felt that those patients whose affect was mobilized would have avoided mentioning or taking up these issues, and some reported that their patients had done just that in other therapies.

The relationship between absence and the nature of the therapeutic alliance was raised by several therapists. One therapist suggested that discussing absences in advance reinforced the therapeutic alliance. Some added here that long absences could be more unworkable than brief absences because some patients could become too self-protective, or too angry or wounded, and unable to tolerate regression or to uncover feelings. One therapist commented that no absences probably does not help the therapy either. A patient's prior history in therapy was seen as playing a role in his or her response to therapist absences. The following case example illustrates the need to learn about and attend to past history, including the role of both therapist and patient in the interaction. Both can collude to avoid critical issues.

Case 3

Mr. C, a 56-year-old writer, had been in analysis for 4 years when his analyst died suddenly. He had begun the analysis because he was unable to go on book tours or do any of the promotional activities required of him in the course of his career. On each trip he became anxious and often found himself returning home suddenly, not fulfilling his responsibilities. Not much changed during the course of the analysis, but he developed a comfortable and trusting relationship with the analyst. With the sudden death of the analyst he was distraught and sought consultation regarding the advisability of continuing his analysis or entering therapy.

Mr. C decided to enter into a twice-a-week psychotherapy relationship with a therapist who told him at the beginning that she frequently traveled for professional meetings and would make every effort to make up appointments, but that their meeting times would be irregular. Initially, Mr. C was untroubled by this, but over the course of several months he revealed that his prior analyst had never taken a vacation or been away for one session and that the current situation was extremely difficult. He decided, however, that it was important to remain in therapy. Over the course of time, he reported feeling enormous fear and anxiety when the therapist left. He believed that if he was a 'good' patient perhaps she would not go. This fear had been present in his analysis and resulted in the omission of many aspects of his history, including a period of substance abuse. He did not disclose any information that he construed to be negative so that he would not risk abandonment. The absences in this therapeutic relationship proved to be anxiety provoking but productive, and Mr. C slowly began to be able to make the trips that advanced his career.

In discussing phases of therapy it was suggested that early in the process (the first 4 or 5 months), fragile, symptomatic, or very primitive patients react more to an absence and that this reaction is related less to specific transference than to immediate need for support. By the end of the first year, neurotic patients were noted to have an increasing awareness, often to their surprise, of the importance of the therapist. This was exemplified by a patient who talked about being relieved and feeling that the absence was convenient, but who found himself at the therapist's office more than once during the therapist's absence.

One respondent also talked about denial and the amount of work it took to mobilize responses to absences, which in the transference may represent significant losses. This therapist also indicated that there might be a positive effect related to an identification with a therapist who was able to lead his or her own life. The absence may also be a time for the patient to integrate the results of the therapy.

Another respondent noted, "I find it is important to be especially vigilant to pick up on reactions of anger, hurt, etc., because my brief explanation of 'attending a meeting' can be used to rationalize that they shouldn't have negative feelings because I am obviously doing something 'important.'" This respondent also noted that short absences were not a problem because they provoked productive material about separation, trust, and so on, and were not overwhelming. Long absences, however, evoked intense anxiety and could be truly disruptive. Some patients, he noted, are at a place where the absence provokes awareness of significant feelings that can be worked with to great advantage.

The therapist's guilt was considered to be an important variable in the patient's response. The therapist must feel "unguilty" enough to permit the patient to respond. The fantasy that one can be the perfect parent by being there all the time is common among therapists. This issue was also seen as important from the training perspective because beginning therapists must learn to deal with their omnipotence or lack of it. Being there all the time can be a way of resolving the profound sense of inadequacy that beginning therapists often feel. Not trying to be the perfect parent of one's fantasy is enormously difficult.

Some therapists underplayed the significance of their absences, whereas others exaggerated the response and encouraged regression. Interruptions can be used positively by some patients, reassuring them of their ability to survive the therapist's absence and to cope with it or enabling them to trust that the therapist will survive and return. Dependence on therapy and the status of the transference were considered to be critical variables in the patient's response. It was noted that after the therapist leaves, some dependent patients indicate that they feel fine and that they are going to stop treatment. Such patients often cannot handle their anger or acknowledge other feelings. On the other hand, one therapist reported that patients called his answering machine because the recording seemed to be a concrete reassurance of his return. The ability to tolerate and work with patient anger was seen as an important therapeutic as well as training and supervisory issue (because trainees may have special difficulty tolerating patient anger and may collude with the patient in avoiding it).

Fear of abandonment and inability to be angry or to depend on a weak and vulnerable "parent" were seen as important issues for patients. Some therapists felt that their patients gained strength by observing that the therapist returned to work after a serious illness or difficulty. It was experienced by some as an inspiration. Yet it can also be a challenge and a reinforcement of the patient's sense of inadequacy. Identification with the therapist appears to be an important variable in patient response, as is illustrated in the following case example:

Case 4

Ms. D, a 42-year-old schoolteacher, began therapy after a divorce and an extended and bitter custody battle. She had always been a self-contained and rather passive person who was generally seen as accepting and easygoing. Even during the worst of the divorce fight, she maintained her composure and sometimes infuriated those who worked with her because she seemed too compliant. When her therapist had to be absent for a conference for a week, she was very accepting and seemed comfortable with the plans he had made for her to be able to contact a colleague of his if there was an emergency. On his return, she became enraged and for the first time in her life exploded with anger and bitterness. When her therapist became defensive, her anger intensified. She subsequently felt that she had violated her own internal prohibitions and had "hooked up with the wrong therapist." She was unable to resume therapy and requested transfer to another therapist.

Another important consideration that emerged from the study responses was the level of therapist experience. One respondent suggested that the negative effects of leaving occurred mainly when the therapist was inexperienced and more rigid about revealing information. This could prevent the therapist from making independent individual judgments about what was clinically best. Over time, it was felt, therapists learn to recognize which patients need more continuity as well as information from the therapist.

Several respondents indicated that when a patient was not told anything about the whereabouts of the therapist, he or she might have altruistic fantasies about what the therapist was doing. On the other hand, others suggested that a patient might harbor a "conventioneer" fantasy about the raucous good times the therapist was supposedly having. This could be difficult for the therapist to bear.

The therapist's experience with an absence can also be an ambivalent one because of what awaits him or her on return. Although one can feel refreshed and relaxed when coming back from vacation, if a patient had had a crisis during the absence, the therapist may have to deal with the patient's anger. At times the return may require more intensive effort and time to deal with guilty and angry feelings. This may promote regression, and it may be a signal of the patient's inability to tolerate absence.

Although gender and age are often thought to affect responses, few differences were reported that were based on these factors. Some respondents commented that men were less sensitive to separation and less expressive of their feelings about it. One respondent suggested that men are slightly more uncomfortable with and defensive about dependency feelings and appeared to accept absence more easily. With regard to age, one therapist reported, "Overall I think younger patients have more negative responses to my absences, yet they insist on seeing a seasoned and high-profile psychiatrist. My older patients are more accepting and mellow about my time away."

Although not specifically stated by these respondents, some differences may be related to type of therapy (e.g., psychoanalysis, long-term intensive psychotherapy, and short-term therapy). With regard to therapeutic modality, one respondent indicated that group patients seem to be more adversely affected by the disruption of their regular group. Moreover, respondents indicated that absences were more difficult for patients in couples and family therapy than for those in individual therapy.

Change in therapist related to changes in training site or clinical rotations was brought up by only a few respondents, and there was no specific discussion of this issue. As the following case example illustrates, though, these changes can be difficult unless the are understood and explicit plans are made:

Case 5

Ms. E, a 29-year-old graduate student with a borderline personality disorder who had made frequent suicide attempts, was seen over the course of many years by a succession of residents in training. Although she initially had difficulty with the changes in residents from year to year and was hospitalized with each changeover, this pattern altered over time. Her therapists learned very quickly that contracted calling times could reduce her hospitalizations and suicide threats. She made slow progress toward independence and was hospitalized less frequently over ensuing years.

"Are You Selective in Taking Patients Into Therapy Because of Anticipated Absences?" (e.g., Not Taking Seriously Ill Patients, etc.)?

Most of the respondents indicated that they were selective in taking patients into therapy, although not necessarily because of their absences. Very disturbed, needy, and borderline patients were seen as most vulnerable to negative reactions to interruptions. Several therapists indicated that suicidal and depressed patients were particularly affected by absences. In general, however, most therapists agreed that their patients seemed to handle absences better than they had thought they would.

Most of the respondents saw few of these more difficult patients, although they stated that this was more often determined by their practice and training preference than by the issue of absence. Only two therapists stated that they did not use their absence as a criterion for patient selection.

One consequence of absences was the need to discontinue therapy. This was viewed as a more likely possibility with borderline patients. One respondent suggested that some patients could not deal with the narcissistic injury of being less important than other commitments and that this could be unworkable. Some patients, it was noted, were more willing to put up with absences for what could be seen as more conventional reasons, such as family commitments, but career demands could raise other issues such as competitive feelings.

CONCLUSIONS

There appears to be some consensus on how to approach therapist absence, and most therapists appear to find solutions that they believe are beneficial for patients. These solutions generally include providing information, when asked, without extensive detail, and maintaining some contact when absences are long. Therapist flexibility also appears to be important.

Although some absences can be seen as beneficial to the patient, this can also be a rationalization. There are no data to support or reject this position. Patients may benefit from absences when they see themselves functioning independently. This can enhance their self-esteem. The necessity to deal with issues of separation, abandonment, and dependency can promote further therapeutic work. Patients who are acutely ill and need active and constant attention, or those who are potentially suicidal, homicidal, or dangerously impulsive, may be in a precarious position when the therapist is absent. Although we can select patients and plan to some extent, our work is not always predictable or controllable.

Consistency and regularity are important aspects of the alliance and the transference, but they are not absolutes. Most experienced therapists feel a sense of responsibility and continuity with patients that keeps them involved even when they are absent. The fact that therapists did report a change in their views about absence and disclosure over time suggests that they may be increasingly comfortable with this aspect of their work or less fearful of being criticized.

Therapist guilt is an important factor in how absence and disclosure is seen and handled. Therapists often feel guilty about abandoning patients or being judged as noncaring or inadequate. They are fearful of being criticized by their colleagues as well as by patients, and they often find it difficult to tolerate patient anger and rejection. On the other hand, hiding behind the rules may reflect insecurity or even discomfort with the kind of intrusion on personal life and space that goes with long-term commitment to clinical responsibilities. The therapist, no matter how much a shadow figure, lives in a kind of fishbowl and is vulnerable. These aspects of the countertransference must be part of the therapist's awareness. To see a patient do well can be gratifying or painful; it can cause therapists to feel successful or less needed in ways that are not so different from the ways parents feel. In either case, our own omnipotence must be tempered by our respect for the patient's autonomy and independence from us. It is critical that the therapist be undefensive and comfortable, understanding his or her motivation both for absence and for disclosure.

REFERENCES

Abend S: Serious illness in the analyst: countertransference considerations. J Am Psychoanal Assoc 30:365–369, 1982

Chernin P: Illness in a therapist: loss of omnipotence. Arch Gen Psychiatry 33:1327–1328, 1976

Dahlberg CC: Perspectives on death, dying and illness while working with patients. J Am Acad Psychoanal 8:369–380, 1980

Dewald P: Reactions to the forced termination of therapy. Psychiatr Q 39:102–126, 1965

Dewald P: Forced termination of psychoanalysis. Bull Menninger Clin 30:98–110, 1966

Dewald P: Serious illness in the analyst: transference, countertransference, and reality responses. J Am Psychoanal Assoc 30:344–363, 1982

Eissler KR: On the possible effects of aging on the practice of psychoanalysis. Psychoanal Q 46:182–183, 1977

Flaherty A: Self-disclosure in therapy: marriage of the therapist. Am J Psychother 33:442–452, 1979

Gitleson M: The emotional position of the analyst in the psycho-analytic situation. Int J Psychoanal 33:1–10, 1952

Givelber F, Simon B: A death in the life of a therapist and its impact on the therapy. Psychiatry 44:141–149, 1981

Hannett F: Transference reactions to an event in the life of the analyst. Psycho-
    anal Rev 36:69–81, 1949

Keith C: Multiple transfers of psychotherapy patients. Arch Gen Psychiatry
    14:185–189, 1966

Kriechman A: Illness in the therapist: the eyepatch. Psychiatry 47:378–386, 1984

Nadelson C, Notman M, Aarons E, et al: The pregnant therapist. Am J Psychi-
    atry 131:1107–1111, 1974

Pumpian-Mindlin E: Comments on techniques of termination and transfer in a
    clinic setting. Am J Psychother 12:455–464, 1958

Reider N: A type of transference to institutions. Bull Menninger Clin 17:58–63,
    1953

Rosenbaum M: Premature interruption of psychotherapy: continuation of con-
    tact by telephone and correspondence. Am J Psychiatry 134:200–202, 1977

Weiner MF: Self-exposure by the therapist as a therapeutic technique. Am J
    Psychother 26:42–51, 1972

Weiss S: The effect on the transference of "special events" occurring during
    psychoanalysis. Int J Psychoanal 56:69–75, 1975

Chapter 5

Countertransference and Divorce of the Therapist

Keith H. Johansen, M.D.

The psychiatric literature contains many references to the countertransference phenomena that occur in psychotherapy during a patient's divorce. Although divorce among the general population and among psychotherapists must have similar incidence, reference to the countertransference that may arise when the therapist is involved in a divorce is absent. In this chapter, I address the countertransference experiences inherent in psychotherapy when the therapist is divorcing.

DEFINITION

For the purpose of this discussion we will not need to resolve the long-standing conceptual controversies over the definition of *countertransference*. Commonly, differences occur along two lines. In one group, the conception of countertransference holds to a strict definition denoting the therapist's conscious and unconscious response to the patient's transference. In a second group, the definition is less strict and includes the therapist's responses to the patient, even when they arise out of the therapist's past and are unrelated to the patient's transference. The question of whether either type of countertransference has constructive value during therapy or is problematic and obstructive of the work to be done has become a part of the controversy involved in these two definitions.

A third definition of countertransference, which is employed with increasing frequency in the literature and which I use in the following discussion, includes all of the emotional reactions of the therapist toward the patient. In this definition, the emotions may arise from any source. This definition avoids the controversy that need not be resolved here and allows the inclusion of material that arises separate from the

patient but will strongly influence the emotional response of the therapist to the patient (Altshul and Sledge 1989).

Although countertransference, however defined, is far too complex
to be reduced simply to a question of whether it is helpful or not helpful, there is an overall tendency among clinicians to view it as an unwanted weakness of emotional strength or maturity on the part of the
therapist. Indeed, we teach our students to watch for the development
of the transference and to be on the lookout for countertransference.
Teachers discuss ways to enhance the growth of the transference but
not that of the countertransference. Thus even in those camps in which
countertransference is viewed conceptually as one more set of data that
can help the therapist understand the patient and the process of therapy, it is not seen as a force to be enhanced as part of the therapeutic
technique.

DYNAMICS OF DIVORCE AS A PROCESS

Divorces differ. Some (probably the minority) appear to pass quite
quickly and with a minimum of turmoil; most are very emotionally
painful and disruptive experiences. Exploring the common dynamics
and change found in many individual cases helps us gain some understanding of this painful experience and predict some of the responses
of the therapist who is caught in this struggle.

Although in common parlance the dissolution of a marriage is often
called "getting a divorce," it is a process that cannot be gotten, obtained, or possessed. Rather, it is complex and involves many individuals over an extended period of time. The process begins long before
any legal papers are served and extends far past the final court-ordered
decree. It is intensely personal to those involved, but it also has a very
public and legal arena. Any divorce is, with possible rare exceptions, a
very painful and stressful experience to many people.

The process of divorce begins privately as one of the marriage partners becomes aware of his or her accumulating doubts about the relationship. Often these are questions about the wisdom of having chosen
a particular spouse or the value of continuing a relationship that is becoming less and less satisfactory. Because these problems and dissatis-
factions have not been resolved within the marriage, a greater distance
develops between the two partners. As they pull away from each other
they may engage in overt fighting of increasing frequency and severity
or silent and incommunicative withdrawal or invest energy and emotions in extramarital preoccupations that are excessive or otherwise destructive to the marriage.

In this process the private aspect of the dissatisfaction becomes more open and ceases to be a matter for the one partner only. Slowly—or suddenly—it becomes an issue for both partners and soon thereafter for other family members as well. At some point, one or both spouses take direct action to move it into the public arena by filing petition for divorce proceedings in public court. The private process of two people's becoming strangers then becomes a community event as well.

This process is not unlike a depiction of falling in love (only in reverse). In that case two strangers meet. One or both realize privately that they feel an attraction for the other. Gradually these feelings are shared with the other, then with family or friends, and finally with the community through a public announcement of engagement or commitment. The two of them begin to think of themselves, and they are thought of by the community, as a couple. In reverse fashion, the filing of a divorce petition in court is a parallel to the public announcement of an engagement. Just as an engaged couple must accomplish much emotional work between the engagement and the day of marriage, so there is a huge emotional and legal task to be completed between the time of filing for divorce and the final decree. Further, just as the marriage ceremony does not create a marriage but only brings about the personal and community setting in which the couple may, through time, effort, and devotion, bring about an actual marriage, so the divorce decree does not create a divorce but merely sets the context in which the two people and the community will know them to have become strangers (Johansen 1980).

Although analogies between becoming a couple and becoming strangers further our understanding of the process, the processes have a different impact on all who are involved. Both marriage and divorce can be vehicles of personal growth, of healing old wounds, and of completing emotional tasks previously left undone, but there the similarities end. Marriage is seen consensually by the individuals and by the community as positive; time-honored rituals support its progress, and the participants are congratulated. Marriage is stressful at times, but the stresses are expected parts of the rites of passage and are met with a sense of optimism and gain. The community participates and resents being excluded from it.

The stresses of divorce are very different. No matter how constructive it is seen to be intellectually, both the individuals and the community struggle with feelings of failure. Rising divorce rates are viewed with social concern. There are no time-honored rituals. Community and family support for the separating partners is sporadic and unpredictable, and the general emotional climate is one of loss rather than gain. It is a time of pain and uncertainty.

This stress infiltrates all aspects of the lives of the couple involved. For the divorcing man or woman who, coincidentally, is also a psychotherapist, the infiltration includes the process of psychotherapy. By definition, to the extent that the therapist's personal responses to this pain and stress appear in the ongoing process of psychotherapy, these responses must be considered countertransference. Because both divorcing and conducting psychotherapy are dynamic, evolving, and ever-changing processes, they interact, and the nature of the countertransference and the therapy evolve with each other. Understanding the force of this outside event on the internal process of psychotherapy can begin with an inventory of the ways divorce has impact on any individual involved.

POINTS OF PERSONAL IMPACT OF STRESS ON THE DIVORCING INDIVIDUAL

To understand the pain and stress of divorce, it is useful to separate the experiences into categories or types of responses. However, none of these responses occurs in isolation; they are lived in symphony and influence each other continually.

Physiological Changes

As psychotherapists we seldom think of physiological changes within the therapist except for brief periods of acute physical illness. Even at these times the therapist may miss a day or two of work and then at the next therapy session he or she reflects on the patient's response to the therapist's absence or on the material raised by this momentary interruption of the therapeutic regularity. As noted above, however, the divorce process is not a brief event. The emotional pain and stress are prolonged and are intensified by the uncertainty of not knowing when it will end. This uncertainty intensifies the stress and the physiological responses to it as well.

Common physiological responses to uncertainty include interruptions of the usual patterns of sleep with subsequent daytime drowsiness. Appetite changes may lead to marked increases or decreases in eating. Weight changes are often rather sudden and may feel out of control. These changes in sleep patterns and eating habits have a sudden and direct effect on the therapist's personal sense of well-being and level of energy.

Physiological changes are especially prominent at times when the everyday demands of life are increasingly unpredictable, and they seem to vary widely with day-to-day events and changes. For example, the duties of life and financial responsibility that had been shared within the marriage become individual responsibilities and must be squeezed into an already unsettled and overloaded schedule of time, budget, and energy. New demands such as meetings with attorneys or awkward social invitations become causes of anxiety and may be anticipated with considerable dread. Consequently, concentrating on day-to-day tasks becomes increasingly difficult.

During a therapy session the therapist's concentration may wander frequently. Maintaining an evenly hovering attention may become a burden or, at times, an impossibility. What will be the source of the energy necessary to meet these demands when the therapist's personal energy level feels depleted? Where will the reserves be found? Some days go much better than others, and the personal physiological changes diminish. But a later day brings new surprises and new demands so that the sense of the unpredictable becomes chronic and insinuates itself into even the quieter days. That physical illness has an increased incidence during this time is not surprising. The impact of divorce on the physical health of the participants is probably second only to the stress of the death of a spouse or child (Holmes and Rahe 1967).

Intrapsychic Changes

The stresses occurring during the period of divorce often become challenges to the individual's intrapsychic structure, even though it had previously attained a dependable degree of stability. Meeting these challenges can lead to growth or regression. In either case, however, it is a time of uncertainty and discomfort.

An intrapsychic area that is almost certain to be caught in the forces of the process is the therapist's self-image. The individual's self-image is very likely, for example, to be caught up in the old question of "Who left whom?" In each instance much is made of being the spouse who left, as opposed to being the spouse who felt left and abandoned. Clinicians know well that the dynamics of a marriage in disarray are never as simple as implied by the stereotyped roles of the one "who leaves the marriage" or the one "who is left." In the earlier stages of the process, however, each of the estranged spouses invariably assumes one of these roles. The effect on each person's self-image is quite different depending on the role assumed. Thus the one who leaves carries a sense of action for which he or she feels accountable. As the pain and disruption seem, at least superficially, to be a consequence of that action, feelings of guilt ensue.

The one who feels left begins to question the type of person he or she is and often begins to doubt self-images that heretofore had supported feelings of self-esteem. The one who assumes the role of being left inevitably struggles with some feelings of abandonment, worthlessness, and depression. This person is more likely to question his or her intrinsic attractiveness as a companion. Traits and self-images that were previously regarded with pride are now in doubt. Reasoning about self-image slips into generalizations such as the idea that because "this spouse finds me unworthy or unattractive then I am."

It is notable that in the assumption of either role, self-image and self-esteem are likely to diminish during the early stages of the divorce process. Self-image and, consequently, self-esteem usually must sustain an attack from another quarter as well. This has to do with loss, the vulnerability to further loss, and the feeling of being helpless to do anything about it.

Most people entering the divorce process anticipate certain losses primarily as they center around the spouse. These include the loss of companionship, confidence, support, and home life as it formerly existed. No matter how sophisticated a person is, however, it would be difficult to anticipate the myriad of day-to-day losses that follow and the emotional weight they accumulate over time. Examples include loss of a routine in daily life, the loss of friends who either attempt to avoid the whole conflict or seem to side with the estranged spouse, and the loss of the understanding of the children, who seemed to appreciate the need for change intellectually, but who now must deal with their own anger, guilt, or resentments. Some of these losses were not expected. The feelings of frustration over these losses, the failure to anticipate them or stop them as they occur, and the ensuing sense of vulnerability to more losses create a self-image of helplessness, where previously a sense of self-confidence and adequacy had become dependable. The rapidity with which these changes occur adds further weight to the power of this dynamic. These pressures on the individual's self-image and subsequent self-esteem have significant influence on the process of psychotherapy.

Interpersonal Changes

Intrapsychic changes cannot be separated from those changes we categorize as interpersonal, but to appreciate the many interrelated facets of this complex process a shift of focus can prove useful. Few aspects of the social structure of any culture play a greater part than family structure in weaving the fabric of people-to-people interaction. Each culture sets forth well-defined, commonly understood, and somewhat rigid rules of who can relate to whom and with what privileges. The social structure depends on commonly recognized roles within the family (e.g., spouse, parent, sibling, and in-law) and within the extended family community. The community has great interest and emotional investment in this structure and in the manner in which it is maintained.

For example, state laws regulate the distribution of assets at the time of death and define the benefits concerning illness or tax obligation that accrue to specific family members, depending on their specific role within the family. The state declares what will be accepted as a valid family unit and how it can be attained (e.g., marriage, common-law marriage, and more recently an interdependent and stable relationship abiding under one roof). No culture can be defined without defining the expected norms of family. Each individual within that culture must recognize and follow the rules or carry the stigma of not doing so (e.g., the illegitimate child who has no state right to inheritance). Within this context we must attempt to understand the long-held social stigma of divorce and its impact on social structure, which extends far beyond the two people participating directly. The first level of organization is thus the family, and from there to the community as a whole, and finally to the state.

When a divorce is no longer contained by differences within the dyad and begins to erupt within the nuclear family, a great sense of uneasiness prevails throughout. The free flow of interaction at all levels of the family no longer has the previously dependable structure to direct and support it. Parents or siblings of the divorcing couple who had lived by the community rules that brought these two families together no longer know what their roles should be. Who can talk to whom and about what? Sides are taken, awkwardness follows, and blaming seems inevitable. Blame must have a culprit, so each faction begins the search for evidence that will relieve them of the burden and stigma of thwarting society's rules of family structure and place it elsewhere. Myths of the two families are brought into play, and differences between the two families that were irreconcilable, but had been ignored by following the structure of family roles, become points of contention. For example, "We've never had a divorce in our family" or "Our family never trusted that fellow—he's a black sheep" are family myths that become very divisive when the structure of family interaction no longer defines family expectation over time.

As the disruption moves out into the greater community, it frequently settles into the institutions of religious communities, schools, or corporate businesses. Each religious group can be defined, in part, according to the rules by which a family may be formed or dissolved. This definition is so strict for some that ignoring the rules leads to expulsion from the religious community. For others, the rules are less strict, but challenges to the norms of the religious community do not go unnoticed, and they must have explanations adequate to satisfy that religious group.

Although less well defined by creed or tenets of faith, community institutions such as schools or corporate business may bring pressure to bear on any individual who appears to tamper with society's rules for family. For example, innuendoes about each divorcing parent's ability to be a good parent are common gossip among teachers and at parent-teacher associations and place great pressure on the divorcing couple. The fabric of society seeks stability, and divorce is seen as a threat to that structure. The social pressure resists dissolving a family (marriage). The same pressure frequently emerges in the work place. Here the sanctions take the form of promotions that are deferred, a wage raise that is withheld, or a job that is actually lost. The firm's rationalization is that the employee is unstable or of questionable judgment. Fellow employees may distance themselves from the person divorcing to protect themselves from the stigma or to enforce society's relentless expectation of the rules of family continuity.

The interpersonal disruption apparent during divorce is seen even at the state level in the child custody laws that regulate some or all aspects of interaction between parent and child after the divorce. A divorce—which is between the parents—costs each of them their heretofore legal right to custody of their own children. After the divorce decree is final, the custody of the child is taken by the state and is held there until the child reaches the age of majority. It is returned to one or both parents only on the basis of a temporary assignment. Thus the legal intervention into interpersonal activity is not only between the estranged spouses; it also invades and limits interaction between parent and child.

The influence these interpersonal disruptions have on the intrapsychic self-image and self-esteem of the individuals cannot be missed. In cyclic fashion, these threats to self-image also impinge on that person's ability to conduct ongoing interpersonal relationships and to meet specific demands at times of intense interpersonal awkwardness or apprehension. Physiological stress, intrapsychic changes, and interpersonal disruptions occur simultaneously and have continual influence on each other. The participant's view of the world changes. Nothing seems quite the same or fits together in the old familiar ways. No longer a member of the world of married men or married women, the divorcing persons feel thrust back to a world of singles, divorced and without partners. Small but persistent reminders of the change are unsettling, such as the common experience of designating ourselves as married, single, or divorced on application forms. And the world has a changed view of that individual.

Effects of the Dynamics of Divorce on the Process of Psychotherapy

With this cursory inventory of the multifaceted effects that divorce has on the individual involved, let us consider the ways in which they may operate within the individual who, coincidently, is also a therapist. What happens within the therapist during therapy is different from what would take place if divorce were not part of his or her life outside therapy. The focus is on material that arises from the world outside therapy and enters the therapy through the therapist, not through the patient. Thus the opportunity for countertransference, as defined above, arises as these externally stimulated feelings are introduced into the process of psychotherapy and toward the patient.

Physiological State of the Psychotherapist

No therapist works as well when he or she is tired or in marginal health. A general sense of physical well-being, together with an expectation of having the energy necessary to complete the therapeutic work, is a substrate or foundation underlying the psychotherapy process. It is a given that allows a sense of confidence about the present and, especially even more important in therapy, a confidence about the future. This quiet expectation about the future, positive in nature but not forcefully stated, is an essential ingredient in the process of therapy and is supplied by the therapist when the patient is unable to do so. It is a lending of the therapist's ego to the patient during treatment.

Chronic fatigue, the loss of energy that accompanies prolonged interruption of sleep, and changes in appetite take a toll on the therapist's sense of optimism about the possibility of change. He or she becomes much more vulnerable to the patient's sense of pessimism about the possibility of change and easily identifies with the patient's doubts. The therapist may then be tempted to join the patient's resistance rather than to analyze it. It certainly seems less demanding at moments when little energy is available to the therapist. The cynicism that follows easily undermines the patient's efforts to change. All of this can easily operate at an unconscious level for both patient and therapist.

Physiological stress, especially when accompanied by poor sleep patterns, also interrupts the therapist's ability to sustain concentration. Listening becomes much more concrete, and the sounds heard by the "third ear" are missed. The whole process of therapy then drifts in the direction of concrete operations (e.g., explaining reality to the patient rather than exploring the metaphor contained within it). This inclination is especially strong within the therapist during peaks of stress when he or she is preoccupied with an anticipated event, such as meeting with a lawyer, or is in the midst of an acute conflict with the children or even the estranged spouse. The therapist may feel that he or she does not have much ego to lend at such times.

Intrapsychic Changes in the Therapist

As noted above, self-image is an intrapsychic structure that is stressed during the process of divorcing. The necessary attributes of a healthy self-image for a therapist are difficult to define, but certainly they include an image stable and predictable enough to serve as an anchor for objectivity. The therapist must be aware of his or her place on the road between subjectivity and objectivity, whereas the patient may get lost in the midst of his or her transference experiences.

Self-image also plays a part in providing the normal supply of narcissism to the therapist. A healthy narcissism, derived over time, accumulates from the experience of being a helpful therapist and provides the strength to sustain periods of uncertainty about the progress or technique of therapy. It supports the therapist in the times of isolation and loneliness that are part of being a therapist.

Because some of these aspects of self-image are under strain or eroded during a divorce, the therapist may feel lost and doubt his or her objectivity. Questions of technique seem more difficult to answer, and mistakes that become apparent to the therapist can no longer be absorbed into the bin of accumulated experience. Instead, they become indications for self-doubt and further questioning. Trainees in their early student years of doing psychotherapy often feel that all they can do is to act like a therapist in the hope that somehow this will suffice until they become what they imagine a therapist to be. This description matches the experience many therapists describe during a divorce. The image of being a therapist fades into the feeling of acting like a therapist, and the therapist is not quite capable of regaining the more secure and satisfying self-image of earlier times.

A quality that many patients bring to therapy is a deep conviction of their helplessness. It is a conviction that the therapist must understand and, at times, experience through the projective identifications of the patient. The therapist's own position on the helpless-adequate scale will be crucial to his or her meeting this aspect of the therapeutic task. The divorcing process exaggerates the therapist's difficulties in this area as he or she lives through the helplessness of limiting the many losses that accrue as it proceeds. The therapist's own experience of being helpless to control the extent and type of losses constitutes a fertile field into which are planted the projections of the patient's feelings of helplessness.

Even more immediately, the therapist feels helpless to defend against the derogatory material the patient may direct toward him or her when the therapist's divorce becomes known to the patient. The therapist is always relatively helpless to control the type of material the patient presents in therapy. Under usual circumstances, this is not a problem, but an important and necessary part of therapeutic technique. Even in relatively small psychiatric communities, such as those many small cities or university settings provide, when the patient learns some incidental fact about the therapist's life and brings it into the session, the material is simply cause for exploration and seldom stimulates the therapist's defensiveness. When the patient makes accusations or raises issues of blame or guilt over which the therapist is already struggling, however, he or she may feel a strong need to correct the patient's image of him or her as a person. This is especially true in the light of the therapist's ongoing effort to maintain a positive self-image. Technique and appropriate conduct of therapy prohibit the therapist's defending himself or herself, but the feelings of frustration and helplessness arise nonetheless.

Often the therapist would like to simply exclude this material from therapy in order to reduce the level of stress and preoccupation. The therapist may respond to these countertransference experiences by attempting to preclude unwanted material from the session, by trying to deal with the "reality" of the situation on an explanatory rather than on an exploratory basis, or by becoming angry and derogatory to the patient in return. Even the well-trained therapist may recognize these "mistakes" of conduct only after they have occurred. This experience then raises questions in the therapist's mind about his or her impulse control.

Countertransference issues of impulse control incorporate aspects of self-image as well as questions of adequacy. The principle of controlling impulses and delaying gratification is at the heart of the process of psychotherapy. Both the patient and the therapist may expect the therapist to exemplify this principle in therapy and in his or her personal life. Any deviation from that principle as evidenced by the therapist's actions is seen by the patient and felt by the therapist as placing in doubt the therapist's capability for the role. The therapist feels a further attack on his or her self-image and in the frustration and low energy reserve of the time often feels helpless to stop these indiscretions of technique. The patient asks, "If you can't get your own life together, why do you think you can help me with mine?"; the therapist privately feels the same thing and feels helpless to change it. The defensiveness and/or anger that follows can easily be directed toward the patient whose remarks are felt to be the cause of all this difficulty. In extreme cases, the therapist rationalizes a way to terminate the patient's treatment in an effort to be rid of the painful experience of hearing this material in therapy.

Interpersonal Countertransference Stimuli

Although therapy presumes an isolated and confidential setting, actually the context is much more public. Each of the participants brings his or her particular context to this mutual setting. On the patient's part are all of the family and friends who know or carefully act as if they do not know that the patient is in therapy. The patient discusses the reasons for seeking help in the first place and often shares experiences with others who have been in therapy or who think they should be. The therapist may have been the subject of lengthy discussions in some of these settings in which many doubts and expectations were aired.

At the same time, although the therapist guards the confidentiality of the patient carefully, the therapist's occupation is known in his or her own community. Family and friends have their own fantasies about what being a therapist is like and their expectations of what attributes of maturity and wisdom therapists should possess. Each therapist establishes a reputation among peers for skill and capability. Being a therapist is a role established by the social community, and those who occupy it must live within its norms. As with all social roles, deviation from the norm brings about the community sanction of stigma.

In the usual setting of therapy these two contexts meet in such a way as to support or even enhance the positive aspects of each. The patient generally selects a therapist whose reputation in his or her community seems to offer the type of help being sought. Friends, family, the clergy, or a personal physician is consulted in making this choice. Naturally, those consulted occasionally ask if the choice worked out well or inquire about the general progress of therapy. Society has a way of monitoring the roles it assigns. At the same time, the therapist receives promotions in an academic setting, is elected to a professional organization or office, or receives the peer recognition accompanying research or a publication. The two contexts are mutually enhancing to the extent that each is known to the other.

In the context of social rules for the formation of a family (marriage), divorce disrupts the mutual enhancement of the two contexts as they overlap in psychotherapy. Patients, family, friends, and referring physicians all raise an eyebrow at the news that the therapist is getting a divorce and question the therapist's ability to help others and the wisdom of continuing therapy with him or her. They may think that the therapist is having a "mid-life crisis" and that treatment should be discontinued "for now," that possibly he or she will be too "upset" to be objective or too preoccupied with the difficulties of divorce to think the patient's problems are important. Patients may fear that talking to the therapist about their own marital difficulties will just be an unwanted burden. Patients' unconscious fantasies may be even more frightening, including ideas such as the possibility that now the therapist is really available as an object for the patient or that the therapist will now want the patient to solve his or her marital difficulties as the therapist did and get a divorce too.

Ironically, the therapist's community may bring even crueler pressures to bear. Peers raise questions about the therapist's stability. Is the divorce a manifestation of a breakthrough of impulses? Is he or she acting out some unconscious conflict that should have been resolved in earlier personal analysis? Should a promotion be withheld or an office or tenure delayed? The therapist's family may feel disillusioned about the wisdom and stability that had been projected on the therapist. Many people (professional colleagues, lay friends, or family alike) come forth with unsolicited advice and criticism. Everyone becomes an expert on the therapist's personal life. Again, it is evidence of society's monitoring the roles it assigns, this time from the therapist's public context.

The interaction of these two worlds as it occurs in therapy is thus the stimulus for considerable transference and countertransference. One of the most vivid examples of this can be seen when a patient brings in material—real, fantasied, or distorted—of what people in the therapist's community are reported to have said about the therapist's divorce. A patient's report that his or her family is questioning the therapist's current state of sanity is painful and difficult for the therapist, but chances are that the therapist deals with most of that in a manner that is ultimately useful to the patient.

When the material is very derogatory and is purported to have been said by the therapist's colleagues, however, the therapist has a much harder time of it. Now he or she feels personally attacked in a manner that is unexpected, and often it comes from a source in which support had been anticipated. Not being able to respond to the patient, to set the record straight, or to ask more about the source and the context of the reputed remark can be extremely frustrating to the therapist and further enhance his or her feelings of helplessness—helpless to do anything about the damaged reputation in the professional community. Certainly the therapist cannot go to the source of the purported derogatory remarks to dispute them or to vent the anger and frustration. The therapist can only deal with the feelings internally: not the ideal way to create a neutral setting in which the therapist can hold an appropriately distant position from the patient's id, ego, and superego, let alone from his or her own intrapsychic structures.

In such a situation, the therapist is much more vulnerable to acting out his or her intrapsychic conflicts through the patient and through identifications with the patient's conflicts. This type of countertransference problem can arise, especially when the patient is playing out his or her own unconscious conflicts through current marital problems. Examples of this countertransference include the following dangers:

➤ The therapist supports the patient's impulse to get a divorce as a way of unconsciously justifying his or her own decisions or as a way of undoing the therapist's fear of losing impulse control.
➤ The therapist identifies with the partner of the same sex in the patient's marital conflict and sees the other spouse in the role of the therapist's own estranged spouse.
➤ The therapist's solutions to marital strife may be imposed on the patient and his or her spouse.
➤ The therapist may act out the guilt he or she is feeling over the divorcing and attempt to "punish" the same sex patient or to favor the opposite sex patient.
➤ The therapist who nourishes a fantasy of being divorced but, for whatever reason, has not done so may encourage patients to seek divorce or, conversely, chastise a patient who tries to explore divorce as a resolution to marital conflict.

Whether such countertransference problems actually develop depends on many factors. First, and by far most potent, is the therapist's intrapsychic strength and structure at the outset. This is true of any countertransference problem, but in any individual instance concurrent factors often serve to increase or decrease the stress placed on the therapist's emotional strengths. These external circumstances are chance factors, such as the age and sex of the patient and the age and sex of the therapist.

Not to be overlooked are the many circumstances in which the therapist is able to guard against these pitfalls but is blamed for them anyway by peers who, out of their own needs, are eager to assume society's role of policing and stigmatizing those who deviate from the expected norms. Actual acting out is very different from being falsely accused of doing so, but either can become very destructive to the process of therapy.

Place of Countertransference in Psychotherapy

Given the process of divorce and such threats to the process of psychotherapy, what can be done to protect the work of therapy, protect the trust and security of the patient, and promote the growth of both the patient and the therapist? Within therapy the growth and progress of the patient must be held as the primary objective around which treatment strategy and decisions are made. In the particular situation we are exploring, however, the therapist is also in emotional pain and in most cases is also attempting to grow during a period of personal crisis. It is important that the process of psychotherapy not be obstructive to that effort either. These two caveats, helping the patient and protecting the therapist, cannot be mutually preclusive if therapy is to continue successfully.

As Charlton (1980) noted, divorce is a psychological experience. When the patient is considering or processing a divorce, a great many transference experiences are subsequently expected to evolve. When the therapist is getting a divorce we can expect countertransference experiences to appear in the same manner. The question then is not whether countertransference experiences will arise, but which ones, when, and with what changes over time. A second question is what to do about them.

The first step in making the countertransference a positive experience must be the acknowledgment that the experience is inevitable. This task will be less difficult if countertransference is approached as being potentially useful and not as a sign that the therapist is beset by pathology, weakness, or moral failure. This acknowledgment must be made as consciously as possible and then faced squarely by the therapist.

This self-confrontation is personally difficult and can be very anxiety provoking to the therapist. No matter how well the therapist is prepared by previous analysis for the therapeutic task of self-monitoring, the continued growth and development of adult life bring new demands and conflicts. These are life experiences that have not been encountered previously. They are part of life's normal progression, which includes aging, children's coming and going in the home, changing financial needs, and the evolving needs (or loss) of one's parents. In some way these events may play some part in the process of divorce and underlie the therapist's participation in them. The tasks of mastering these new developmental junctures are no less imperative than the developmental tasks of childhood. The exploration of these new demands, the conflicts they reawaken, and the defenses that these conflicts stimulate require exploration and resolution in order to assure continued growth and maturation. These conflicted areas may play a significant role in the development of countertransference and, therefore, may be discovered in the therapist's effort to explore his or her ongoing participation in therapy.

Not uncommonly, therapists require help in this self-exploration. The assistance can take as many forms as are dictated by the needs or circumstances of each individual. Talking with friends or peers about their divorce experiences can provide very useful perspectives. Therapists often think of themselves as being less needy than others or fear that if their needs show, especially during a time of crisis, they will be seen as regressing or insufficiently analyzed. The latter criticism often is meant to imply a basic character flaw and is particularly painful to someone who is already feeling vulnerable. Because of these kinds of fears and the doubts about who is a friend or who is critical or sides with the estranged spouse, divorcing therapists may find reaching out to be difficult. This apprehension is often more intense during the early days, when help is most needed.

Consequently, a second option for finding such help may be to arrange for supervision by a respected colleague, on a regular basis, and over such time as is needed to explore the countertransference experiences. Supervision is a time-honored tradition for therapists at many stages in their careers and may be less threatening, especially when a therapist is already feeling quite vulnerable. Supervision can be much more specific than general sharing with friends, and it carries the advantage of maintaining confidentiality for both the therapist and the patient involved.

The tenacity or nature of the conflicts that are discovered beneath the countertransference problems as they are discussed in supervision may prompt the therapist to return to his or her own psychotherapy for brief work. If the therapist can see this as a sign of strength rather than weakness, the results can be very gratifying to the therapist and of great benefit to his or her patients. As we become more aware of the task of continuing to grow throughout adulthood, we may be more free to encourage our patients and ourselves to turn to therapy for brief periods of time when such help would be useful. Each stage of adult life brings new challenges and different requirements for a sense of well-being (Colarusso and Nemiroff 1981; Levinson et al. 1978; Sheehy 1976). As noted earlier, these requirements vary with many factors, such as age, sex, changes in health, or changing configuration of the family. These are signs of growth and activity, not of weakness or pathology. The therapist who hesitates to seek help when feeling lost during the process of therapy or when in doubt about a particular technique may be responding to real forces that are more unconscious than necessary. Exploring this question in supervision or therapy can be very constructive and need not be difficult.

What is different about the countertransference that develops during divorce from that which might follow any major event in the life of the therapist? Is there anything in this particular life occasion that is unique or is similar to any other challenging life event, such as the loss of a child or the development of a debilitating or fatal illness? Aspects that are similar are probably more numerous than those that are unique. An area of similarity can be found in the ongoing sense of vulnerability and helplessness (perceived or imagined) to alter the life event and the resultant anger and frustration that are such a major part of the divorce experience. In each of these life events, such feelings can arise.

Still, when exploring divorce we find that it can be a pivotal point in our understanding of the development of countertransference and in our search for ways to use that awareness to the benefit of the therapy process. Although the nature and intensity of these feelings varies with day-to-day circumstances, such as divorce meetings that must be met and remarks that the children made that morning, the central theme is loss—loss of the spouse, loss of dreams for marriage and life together, loss of a large part of the community that had been shared, loss of the old and expected relationship with the children, and loss of having felt successful as a parent or spouse. Many of these losses are replaced in time. There are new friendships; different, but appropriate relationships with the children; trust in the support of the community; and feelings of confidence and success. These changes do not emerge evenly, and each stage in the process brings new areas in which the therapist feels vulnerable. Just knowing, however, that it is a process, may help the therapist feel more in control. Many of the feelings of vulnerability are responses to external stimuli. These feelings, although having aspects that are similar to many of life's losses, may exhibit some characteristics that are peculiar to the divorcing process.

Another similarity to the feelings that follow the death of a child or a spouse may be the blaming that is so prevalent in divorce. For a period in the mourning process after the death, the parent or spouse asks himself or herself if anything could have been done to prevent the disaster. Self-searching and blame inevitably follow. Some of the blame can be placed, with great anger, on other individuals, such as doctors or other family members, who may have had some part in the event. Self-searching and blaming of others is a common occurrence in divorce also.

Divorce may be unique, however, in its raising the question of impulse control. Any divorce raises questions in the minds of many people having to do with the divorcing individual's stability, patience, or willingness to stay with the marriage long enough to resolve the problems. Not only do the family and community ask these questions, but the persons involved ask themselves or project the blame for the supposed lack of stability and patience onto others. For the person who is also a therapist, such questions take on a particular dynamic quality because questions of stability are translated into doubts about impulse control and the ability to delay gratification. Whether raised by the therapist himself or herself, by colleagues, or by the community, the question has a powerful impact on the intrapsychic and interpersonal dynamics of the divorcing person. Its impact on the countertransference appears to be unique and must be met in any attempt to resolve countertransference issues in a manner that is beneficial to patient and therapist alike.

Safeguards

Clearly the most constructive approach to countertransference phenomena lies in the efforts of the therapist to bring them to consciousness, resolve underlying conflicts, and allow both patient and therapist to go on with the adult task of growth and development. In the meantime, though, there are technical remedies or safeguards that can be supportive to the more definitive work being done. These must be peculiar to each individual, but some general ideas may be useful.

The therapist who is divorcing can be more vigilant about changing outside stimuli that can be changed. For example, in some situations, the impersonal quality of the legal system can be used supportively. Either or both contending parties may elect to leave more of the representation and negotiating to the respective attorneys, thus gaining distance from the conflict at a time when the personal feelings of failure and loss are great. Accepting that which cannot be changed or controlled as part of the usual process of divorce can also be very supportive. A productive stance in the battle against the feeling of vulnerability can be found in the realization that facing a crisis carries the opportunity of growth and change. Countertransference thereby becomes a stimulus for growth, a reminder that hope dwells within crisis, and a benefit to both patient and the therapist.

Other arenas to which the therapist can turn in the midst of the countertransference experiences include those time-honored guidelines that we might call the "techniques" of therapy, which were learned early in training, tested against years of supervision, and modified only slowly with long and carefully considered experience. They are not rigid or universal, but they are developed to fit the particular strengths and style of the therapists using them. They serve as a baseline against which deviations can be detected. In the same way that the legal system might serve to offer some distance and an impersonal stance when useful to the divorce process outside of therapy, so the adherence to familiar and time-tested psychotherapy techniques may make a greater involvement and intimacy tolerable within therapy.

There are two ways therapeutic techniques can be used for this purpose. Both arise as warnings that greater involvement within therapy is at risk of being used to satisfy the countertransference demands of the therapist rather than to facilitate a greater empathy of the patient's feelings and an enhanced intuition of strategy that might strengthen treatment. The first warning comes from the therapist's urge to experiment or to devise a "new" technique because of a belief that this particular case is different or because of the conviction that the therapist's own experience now bestows the ability to understand the emotional pain of the patient much better than can the therapist who has not had a divorce. The divorcing therapist then attempts shortcuts to relieve the pain through direct manipulation, rationalizing that the patient need not suffer through the work necessary to understand the underlying conflicts and defenses. Although, indeed, the therapist may have a greater appreciation of the patient's struggles and pain, that appreciation can be put to better use in helping the patient explore and then resolve his or her conflicts within the guidelines of the usual therapeutic techniques.

The second warning comes as the therapist finds that he or she is having experiences within or about therapy that are different from those that have been established over time. Some common examples include

> The therapist experiences a growing involvement in his or her patient's marital conflict and its outcome. Particularly significant is the realization that this preoccupation extends outside the therapy session itself.
> Persistent rescue fantasies arise toward the patient or spouse. These kinds of thoughts can occur in any psychotherapy process and often allow the therapist to know something about the patient's uncon-

scious wishes or demands. The point here is not that such fantasies occur within the therapist, but that they are experienced with an unusual quality or in an unexpected manner.

➤ The therapist finds himself or herself taking sides in the patient's marital differences. This often takes the form of accepting the patient's stories about the spouse at face value rather than exploring this material in the light of the total work being done and the patient's character and defenses. The therapist identifies with the patient in assigning blame to the absent spouse.

➤ The therapist experiences an urge to give advice or to guide the outcome of an interpersonal struggle the patient is facing. In these situations the therapist may realize a personal feeling of satisfaction as the patient chooses a given course of action—a feeling that it was "right."

➤ The therapist feels annoyed by the patient's discussion of marital or other interpersonal conflicts. This phenomenon may be a global avoidance of the matter or a persistent attempt not to hear the painful affect associated with the material.

➤ The therapist feels the need to share personal experiences with the patient and compare them with the patient's experiences.

In each of these examples, the warning the therapist must hear is not simply that these feelings occur, but that the countertransference feelings arise from present experiences that exist in the therapist's life outside of therapy, that these feelings are being experienced in ways that are unusual and are at risk of being acted out in therapy.

CONCLUSIONS

Divorce is a process that may involve the contemporary psychotherapist as it may any member of society. Often it is a very painful and disruptive time during the life of all individuals involved. The divorce process, in which two married people become strangers, is also a public experience within the matrix of social order and has repercussions in many contexts. The complexity of these personal, social, and state (legal) interactions places great stress on the primary participants. The stresses are both physiological and psychological and inevitably infiltrate all aspects of the participants' lives.

Because psychotherapy is also an emotionally intimate process, no personal stress on the therapist can be ignored during therapy. The feelings toward the patient within therapy that are generated by the divorce outside of therapy are a form of countertransference, and the ways they are experienced and then used must be held accountable to all the usual criteria of good therapeutic practice. The very presence of the countertransference experiences is to be expected, but the obligation rests on the therapist to use them in a way that is supportive of the therapy process and facilitates both the patient's and the therapist's continued growth. Recognizing these countertransference experiences is a primary step toward these goals. The therapist must find a way to face them directly if they are not to develop a life and action of their own. The intense and very painful feeling of vulnerability to continued loss and the sense of helplessness to stop these losses, especially during the early part of the divorce process, engender many self-doubts, personally and professionally, within the therapist. Questions of the therapist's impulse control and ability to delay gratification must be kept within a constructive perspective and not become excuses for derogatory responses on the part of the therapist and/or his or her peers.

Although sharing these experiences with supportive friends may provide sufficient help, the most efficient resolution is often gained from direct psychotherapy supervision or personal psychotherapy. The many losses can be replaced in time by growth, personally and professionally. In the long run the patient will benefit from this renewal also if the countertransference has not been used destructively in the meantime.

There is a tendency on the part of the lay public to idealize the role of the therapist. Therapists, as clinicians, have some understanding of that. If, however, as an individual, the therapist begins to believe that idealization, his or her patient will be in trouble. The therapist who is in the midst of the divorcing process responds just as any other person in pain and must make adjustments and tend to his or her needs as would anyone else. Expecting more of oneself creates a very lonely situation filled with disillusionment that ultimately damages the patient.

REFERENCES

Altshul VA, Sledge WH: Countertransference Problems, in American Psychiatric Press Review of Psychiatry, Vol 8. Edited by Tasman A, Hales R, Frances A. Washington, DC, American Psychiatric Press, 1989, pp 518–530
Charlton RS: Divorce as a psychological experience. Psychiatric Annals 10(4):12–21, 1980
Colarusso CA, Nemiroff RA: Adult Development. New York, Plenum, 1981
Holmes T, Rahe R: The social readjustment rating scale. J Psychosom Res 11:213–218, 1967
Johansen KH: Divorce: a process and a stress. Tex Med 76:63–66, 1980

Levinson DJ, Darrow CN, Klein EB, et al: Seasons of a Man's Life. New York, Knopf, 1978
Sheehy G: Passages. New York, EP Dutton, 1976

Chapter 6

When Both Therapist and Patient Are Divorcing: The Role of Supervision

James M. Trench, M.D.

Chapter 5 of this volume focused in illuminating detail on the problems that arise in the course of therapy when the therapist undergoes a divorce. A situation that compounds the difficulties of such cases occurs when the patient, as well as the therapist, is involved in divorce proceedings. In this chapter, based on my experience as the therapist or supervisor of therapists faced with that specific set of circumstances, I deal with the unique transference-countertransference complications that result.

An extensive literature search revealed nothing specifically focusing on the countertransference and transference reactions involved when both therapist and patient are divorcing. This is interesting given the fact that divorce is a common occurrence in the United States. In the 1960s, nearly 33% of all marriages ended in divorce; during the 1980s, approximately 50% of the couples getting married would later separate or divorce (Glaser and Borduin 1986). However, a literature search did reveal reports exploring the therapist in the divorce process and its effects, both personally and professionally. One article (Pappas 1989) noted that nearly one-third of therapists interviewed were distressed about personal marital problems and divorce; another (Norcross and Prochaska 1986) stated that therapists experience marital problems and divorce at a rate equaling or exceeding that of the general population.

In this chapter, the countertransference issues that develop as a result of both therapist's and patient's being involved in divorce are explored from several perspectives: my personal reactions as I and my patients concurrently struggled with the emotional and legal realities of marital separation and divorce; my reactions as supervisor to other therapists who were in the midst of divorce and treating patients in similar circumstances; and the reactions of a therapist who was my patient and was involved in a divorce while treating a divorcing patient.

The observations and conclusions presented here are based on a review of the case histories of patients in the 1960s who were going through divorce and the extensive records of their therapists, who themselves were personally involved in divorce. Observations have been drawn from the direct contact between my patients and myself as a therapist, from the indirect contact with a patient in my role as a supervisor and then therapist of a colleague, and from the indirect contact with patients as a supervisor of eight other therapists. Within this group of 10 therapists (including myself) are represented 50 patients, all of whom were either considering divorce, in the process of divorce, or in the stage following divorce.

ANATOMY OF DIVORCE

To understand more fully the multiple dynamics that take place between a therapist and a patient simultaneously involved in divorce, it is important to understand the process of divorce and the stages of loss involved and to evaluate which phase of separation or loss is present. Pappas (1989) described four stages of loss: stage I, shock or denial; stage II, protest; stage III, despair; and stage IV, detachment or resolution. In addition, I have defined three phases in the divorce process: in phase I, the individual is considering divorce; phase II is the legal and emotional process of the divorce; and phase III is the period after the divorce. In phase III a distinction is made between "legally divorced" and "emotionally divorced" because, although the individual may be legally separated, he or she may not have achieved emotional separation. The specific countertransference issues presented in the case examples below are determined by both the phase and the stage in which both patient and therapist are each involved (Table 6–1).

THERAPIST AND PATIENT SELECTION PROCESS

Therapist selection did not appear to be random in this review of case histories from the 1960s. Those patients involved in the divorce process stated that because they felt stigmatized by their "marital failure" they looked for a therapist who was, like themselves, also involved in divorce. They believed that a therapist in a similar situation would be less critical and more sensitive to and supportive of their needs. This was particularly true for male patients, who tended to have less general support from friends and colleagues. The women in the group seemed to have better developed support systems, with strong and uncritical support from friends and family, and thus were less concerned with the marital status of the therapist. In contrast, patients (both men and women) who were unaware of the possibility that they were moving toward divorce did not seem to consider the marital status of the therapist as a criterion in their selection.

Two of the therapists made the decision not to treat patients engaged in divorce. Both believed that they would be unable to maintain a "healthy distance" from these patients. However, in general, the therapists were not eager to engage patients involved in marital problems. There were several reasons for this. Despite its increasing occurrence, divorce still carried a stigma. It was easier for a patient to obtain an appointment if he or she was the "victim" of divorce rather than the individual seeking the divorce. Reluctance to engage a divorcing patient also occurred if the therapist was personally involved in a divorce, due to a fear that an overinvolved transference-countertransference reaction through identification, if too intense, could jeopardize treatment rather than help. Another influencing factor was concern that involvement as a therapist would require a consequent legal involvement.

PATIENT DEMOGRAPHICS

Eighty percent of the 50 patients were women, half of whom were in their late forties. Most of these women did not work outside the home, holding instead the traditional job of housewife. The men were career-oriented, driven individuals in their late thirties and early forties. Despite the increasing number of divorces in the early 1960s, the negative societal and familial attitudes toward divorce had a profound effect on those involved in the divorce process. Even when divorce was the only appropriate solution, the negative, unsupporting atmosphere of the times made it difficult for those involved in divorce to effectively toler-

Table 6–1. Anatomy of divorce: stages of loss and phases of a divorce

Loss		Divorce	
Stage	Description	Phase	Description
I	Shock or denial	I	The individual is considering divorce
II	Protest	II	Legal and emotional process of the divorce
III	Despair	III	The period after the divorce
IV	Detachment or resolution		

Source. Stages of loss adapted from Pappas 1989.

ate the process. The reactions of individuals, both male and female, to the social and emotional situations created by the divorce process were in large part determined by their support systems. Indeed, the presence or absence of a strong support network was an important factor in deciding to seek treatment. Women tended to present themselves for treatment when they felt the beginning of loss of support from family and friends. Men tended to seek treatment because, due to a concern about what others would think of them, they often did not develop any support system and felt isolated from others with whom they could share their hurt and rage.

The majority of patients in this study fell into one of the three phases of divorce mentioned above (Table 6–1). The remaining patients approached therapy without any awareness that they were moving toward divorce. The patients who were in the process of divorce could be divided into two groups: those who wanted active treatment, and those who were seeking a psychological navigator to guide them through the perilous straits of the legal process. The latter group needed more counseling than treatment, which would lead to awareness and change.

THERAPISTS AND SUPERVISION

There were two categories of therapist who sought help from another therapist: those who were concerned that their sexual controls were failing sought patient status, and those who were concerned about a variety of countertransference issues, such as inattention, adverse attitudes, and lack of progress in treatment, sought supervision. The therapists who requested only supervision had experienced early warning signs of increased frustration in their professional lives. The most common warning was an awareness of inconsistency between their theoretical orientation and practice, which was often initially rationalized as an innovative approach, until anxiety led the therapist to seek out a colleague for advice.

Some therapists who sought supervision were less troubled by the intensity of the countertransference reaction. They seemed more intellectually aware of the early warning signs of a nontherapeutic relationship and were able to discuss openly their defenses against dependency, hostility, sexual anxiety, overdetachment, and their lack of openness to the patient's desire to discuss a specific divorce situation. These therapists recognized the possibility of an increased affective quality in the treatment process because of the similarity between their situation and that of the patient. With supervision, they were better able to use the countertransference reactions therapeutically.

Other therapists sought supervision because they feared they were becoming "romantically involved" with their patients, and supervision helped them to separate their own divorce issues from the issues of their patients. These therapists often felt victimized and manipulated by their patients with resultant feelings of frustration and anger. They recognized the potential to "act out" during treatment. Although, as discussed below, none of these therapists did act out in any physical or sexual manner, they were troubled by their fantasies and their patients' intense transference reactions.

More antitherapeutic countertransference reactions occurred when both the patient and the therapist were in phase II (the active process) of divorce and in stages II (protest) and III (despair) of loss than in any other set of circumstances. However, troublesome countertransference reactions did occur when the therapist and patient were in different phases, particularly when the patient was further along than the therapist in the divorce process. An antitherapeutic countertransference reaction could also occur when a patient entered into therapy without a conscious awareness of a movement toward divorce, but one developed during treatment. If the patient did not have sufficient ego strength to understand this development to be a result of treatment, it was possible he or she would see it as the therapist guiding him or her toward divorce for personal gain. This could be a perilous situation if the countertransference had been, in fact, provocative.

Perhaps the most difficult issue for many therapists to resolve was the occurrence of a strongly negative countertransference reaction. In this situation, there was a tendency to displace those feelings and attitudes that they considered irreversible from their own personal situation and, as a result, to conclude that negative countertransference reactions were irreversible.

COUNTERTRANSFERENCE ISSUES

Dynamic therapy is never a comfortable situation, but when an inordinate level of discomfort develops, it is a signal that the relationship is becoming problematic. Despite this, all but two therapists in this group were able to continue treating their patients. These two had initially sought supervision from me and then went into intensive treatment where they made the decision temporally not to engage in treatment with divorcing patients. Both felt that they were not able to maintain a "healthy distance" from their patients. This is particularly important with patients who are actively feeling rejected, as in phases I and II of divorce. In phase III, the patient with similar ego strength is beginning to understand his or her own contributions to the marital discord and can tolerate moderate inconsistency on the part of the therapist who is struggling with countertransference issues.

Therapists who become more secure would comfortably question early signs of overinvolvement such as overdiagnosis, defenses against dependency, hostility, sexual anxiety, detachment, and lack of openness. It is clear that when the patient and therapist are concurrently involved in a common problem there is an enhancement of and an increase in the affective quality of the treatment situation. However, there is also the potential for antitherapeutic countertransference reactions to occur. As noted above, the greatest problems occurred when the therapist and patient were in phase II (the active process) of divorce and in stages II and III (protest and despair) of loss.

The concept of countertransference was first elucidated by Freud (1910). He stated that countertransference "arises in [the physician] as a result of the patient's influence on his unconscious feelings" (p. 144). Heimann (1950) defined countertransference as "all the feelings which the analyst experiences towards his patient" (p. 81). She included the unconscious but also focused on another aspect that she called the analyst's "emotional response" to the patient. She also noted that if the analyst allows himself or herself to become aware of this countertransference, the feelings can be used to identify the areas that are significant to the patient at that time. The process whereby such a situation becomes possible can be understood through the concept of projective identification.

The countertransference issues experienced by the therapists become clearer if divided into two types. The first type includes issues perceived to be problems by the majority of therapists; the second type includes those issues that were experienced by certain therapists in specific situations. A general problem area was the premature exploration of the subject of initial attraction to the future spouse. This question usually ushered in self-blame and guilt. The therapists in this group reported intense resistance from patients and a distracting preoccupation within themselves. This countertransference issue was discussed by Bellis (1989), who stated, "We see that there are dangers in both negative and positive transference and countertransference; for idealization is inherent in primitive love. And behind every idealization lurks its antithesis—the well-known devaluation" (p. 62). He further noted that "the dangers of positive countertransference are like dangers of falling in love. We tend to idealize, 'put on pedestals,' our victims and feel ourselves victimized as reality sets in. This setting in of reality is called the disillusioning process and is inherent in both marriage and therapy" (p. 62).

Depression in both therapist and patient was another arena in which antitherapeutic problems arose. Depression in the therapist often led to a passive-detached mode that compounded the patient's depression and guilt, as the lack of responsiveness on the part of the depressed therapist could be interpreted by the patient as indifference. Self-defeating behavior often coupled with depression was prevalent in phase II of divorce and stage III of loss. When therapists and patients were concurrently in this situation, the issues became immense. Case 1, reported by one of the supervisee therapists, illustrates this phenomenon:

Case 1

Mr. A, a 36-year-old businessman, presented himself for treatment with the chief complaint that he was unable to function well at work. Mr. A was in phase II of the divorce process, as was his therapist. Although he usually went through an assessment period of three or four visits with each new patient, the therapist made instead an immediate commitment to see this patient, feeling that Mr. A was losing his last area of proficiency—his abilities as a businessman.

As therapy progressed, the therapist began to find it difficult to maintain his attention and concentration during the sessions. To "protect himself" from these lapses of attention, the therapist increasingly became more passive in the treatment situation. After five sessions, he became aware of the intensity of his feelings when he saw himself as sympathetic rather than empathetic to the patient. Mr. A was acting in a self-defeating manner in many aspects of his life; he had become a compulsive spender and had developed the inordinate need to punish himself in sexual relationships with individuals whom he described as social and intellectual inferiors. The therapist saw both himself and Mr. A becoming increasingly obsessional and perceived the treatment as stalemated.

The therapist sought help and in the process of supervision began to ventilate his own feelings. After two supervisory sessions with me, he recognized that he was having difficulties with more patients than those involved in a divorce process. A decision was made to continue supervision with me but also to enter into treatment with another colleague. With treatment, the therapist became aware of how he was reacting to Mr. A's resistance and found himself able to be more active in confrontation, as well as in the interpretation of issues that arose during the sessions. Supervision and treatment also helped the therapist to distance himself from Mr. A. As a result, new goals of treatment were negotiated and it was decided that Mr. A needed only brief supportive therapy instead of the intensive therapy they had been engaged in. At the same time, the therapist began to reach out for support among colleagues and friends, and, as he developed a support group, his depression gradually lifted.

There is a problem of how much personal information a therapist should spontaneously share with a patient. The majority of patients had some knowledge of the marital situation of their therapists, and this offered a rich field for speculation. There was often concern that the therapists had not been open enough or that they had revealed too much—verging on a confession—to their patients. Responding to the advocates of "clearing the air" by full disclosure, Heimann (1960) pointed out that "a communication of this kind represents a confession of personal matters pertaining to the analyst, and would mean a burden to the patient and lead away from the analysis. Therefore, it should not occur" (p. 12).

I would add that because patients project something they are unable to tolerate, they are likely to experience such a confession as confirmatory evidence that the analyst's projections are intolerable since the analyst is having to get rid of them also. Abend (1982) also addressed the dilemma of how much to tell a patient (in this case about the therapist's illness): "Several were in the field of medicine and . . . those I told what had actually occurred; others, I simply informed that I would fully recover. Those patients to whom I did not tell anything factual did perfectly well. Of those I told, some disbelieved me, others distorted what they noted or what I had said, some complained of being told anything, others about not being told more; in short, each reacted to what I said or did not say in his own way" (p. 374). Abend's message is clear. Transference is usually stronger than reality, and knowing how much to say, how to say it, and under what circumstances is important to understanding and analysis.

The therapists in this group found it helpful to the treatment process to respond to questions such as "Are you separated?" "Are you in the process of divorce?" and "Have you been divorced and have you remarried?" Not to respond was interpreted by patients as an unwillingness to be open. Although the focus of this discussion is on countertransference, it is important to note here that patients will always, as part of their transference reaction, explore these areas either directly or indirectly. It is always better to assume that patients know much more about you than they will communicate. This is particularly true in short-term therapy situations.

CASE EXAMPLES

The following case examples explore the issues regarding how much personal information the patient knows or should know about the therapist's marital situation. In Case 2, the patient focused on an area that was positive in her divorce situation but was a negative issue in the therapist's own divorce, thus causing conflict for the therapist.

Case 2

Ms. B, a 22-year-old junior executive, came to treatment stating that she just needed to talk about many things but that nobody was willing to listen to her. She was in phase III, having been divorced 3 months before coming to treatment. She was still mourning the loss of a very difficult marriage in which there had been considerable physical violence directed toward her, but she had recently begun to reach out toward men. She stated that she did not want to go from the "frying pan into the fire."

Ms. B's therapist reported that Ms. B was a very engaging young woman, intelligent, and psychologically minded. She had no children and had found a responsible job. This was a new situation for her as she had gone directly from high school into a marriage with a man 5 years her senior. She stated that she and her husband had been immediately attracted to each other, and that 2 months after meeting they were married. As she moved along in treatment, she began to uncover the tremendous idealization present in the beginning of her marriage and the subsequent disillusionment that eventually replaced it. Guilty feelings about the failure of her marriage began to surface after the therapist pointed out her tendency to provoke anger. To control these feelings of guilt and to rid herself of feelings of blame, she provocatively pursued the issue of how well she had done in the divorce settlement. She stated further that her friends, as well as her attorney, felt she had done well, indeed, perhaps "too well." The therapist was himself in phase II of divorce and found that this theme of "too well" began to cause him to feel resentment toward Ms. B. Her obsessional management of her guilt was met by his obsessional defense against his rage, and therapy was severely impeded.

To remove this stalemate, the therapist sought supervision, during which several options were discussed. After discussing these options with Ms. B, it was mutually decided that she would not be seen for a month. During this hiatus, the therapist continued in supervision and was soon able to recognize that the patient's statement of doing "too well" had represented a real threat to him because he was involved in a financial negotiation process with his estranged wife. This recognition enabled him to begin to work through his angry feelings.

After a month, Ms. B and the therapist resumed therapy, which in turn took new directions and became more productive. Ms. B was able to confront and work through her need to provoke rage, and the therapist, who had been blinded by her description of being the victim of her former husband's rage, had regained his perspective.

Abend (1986) referred to a similar clinical situation when he wrote that "a compelling need to rescue victims and condemn sadistic fathers, also derived from powerful unconscious forces within the analyst, promoted an identification with the patient that dictated selective interpretation of the victimized stance, and effectively blinded the analyst for a long time to the provocative, masochistic elements in his analysand, despite advice from colleagues regarding the material" (p. 571).

Options as to the depth, length, and frequency of treatment according to the patient's needs should be discussed at the first meeting. A person's needs during the divorce process can vary not only from individual to individual, but within the same individual depending on what stages of loss and phases of the divorce process he or she is in. This determination of treatment type is crucial in helping both the therapist and the patient maintain positive direction. The following case example illustrates this point:

Case 3

Mr. C, a 52-year-old owner of a small business, was seen when he was in phase II–stage II of the divorce process. His therapist, was also in phase II–stage II, which led to an eagerness on the part of the therapist. Mr. C was having fantasies that the divorce would be so devastating that he would lose his business and his friends. He began to hope that he would have a heart attack and die. Early in therapy it became apparent that he was deeply depressed and was unable to visualize any future for himself. He had actively thought about suicide, including what the most successful method would be. He was hospitalized and placed on antidepressant therapy.

The depression began to clear before there could have been any psychopharmacological response, and Mr. C began to become increasingly verbal and productive. The therapist outlined a treatment plan that would include twice-a-week psychotherapy of an in-depth, explorative type, and although Mr. C expressed some reluctance about this plan, he continued with his regularly scheduled appointments. He also continued the antidepressant medication and began to uncover intrapsychic problem areas.

Mr. C felt that he was doing well in therapy, but it was apparent that the rest of his life was becoming a shambles. He had a successful business with which he was preoccupied and for which he was completely responsible. He was unable to delegate any of this responsibility. He was feeling tremendous anger toward his spouse because he knew that the more money he made in his business, the higher the alimony settlement would be. Money was clearly a major issue in this divorce. In spite of these deeper problems, Mr. C made it clear to the therapist that he did not want to engage in intensive therapy at that time. He was encouraged by the psychological insights that he had gained in treatment and felt positive about the treatment situation, but because the rest of his life was suffering he felt he could ill afford to work in treatment to the degree that the therapist wanted. The therapist and Mr. C agreed to four more visits at which time termination of work was begun.

The important element in Case 3 was the therapist's need to treat Mr. C more extensively than he could tolerate. Mann (1984-1985) discussed a similar issue that arises during time-limited psychotherapy: "Therapists may feel frustrated by both the limited goals of brief treatment and by the limitations of time. It is not unusual in discussions about patients treated in some form of brief therapy for questions to be raised as to why this or that conflict or issue was not dealt with sufficiently or at all, as though it is not understood that if a therapy is designated as brief it must follow reasonably that the goals of treatment have been circumscribed" (pp. 205–206). Although Mr. C did not describe frustration at the incompleteness of his treatment, his therapist was feeling frustration from his countertransference perspective. He had not integrated Mr. C's outside pressures into the treatment plan, but had seen instead the patient's potential for in-depth treatment. The therapist's first reaction was frustration with his patient and then awareness of his overly ambitious treatment goal for the patient.

The possibility that a negative countertransference reaction could lead to the overdiagnosis of a difficult patient was another issue that occurred among this group of therapists. The following case explores how this could happen:

Case 4

Ms. D, a 28-year-old housewife in phase I (considering divorce), described symptoms of immobilizing depression, but was nevertheless very engaging in the first two interviews. She discussed being very disillusioned with everyone except her therapist, whom she saw as being extremely helpful. She described her husband as having been a wonderful person until he suddenly turned on her. The husband was threatening divorce, and Ms. D was denying any responsibility for the marital discord. She had become so preoccupied with her present situation that she was unable to give a complete history of her past. She repeated "the past is the past and it is gone and I can't think beyond the present." This cluster of signs and symptoms was not unusual in borderline patients. Ms. D provoked a negative countertransference reaction in the therapist, who stated, "She presented dynamic material, overvalued me, and then proceeded to frustrate efforts to intervene." It was common to explain away negative transferences as inevitable with borderline patients. Ms. D was scheduled for three additional appointments for a more complete evaluation.

By the third appointment there was less focus placed on history taking and more discussion of the "here and now." Ms. D discussed her grandmother, who had always been the stabilizing force in her life (her mother was "bipolar"), and the rage and panic she felt when her grandmother unexpectedly criticized her for her failed marriage. Through discussion, Ms. D became aware that because the grandmother had, herself, coped with an unhappy marriage, the criticism toward her granddaughter was an expression of her rage at her own inability to extricate herself from a difficult marriage. From this point on, Ms. D was able to talk about the future and to begin the process of overcoming the feelings of sadness and anger.

Case 4 illustrates clearly the need to be able to tolerate the initial negative countertransference reaction that can result in overdiagnosis.

OTHER COUNTERTRANSFERENCE ISSUES

There were other problems that arose from countertransference reactions between patients and therapists concurrently involved in the divorce process. Some patients became concerned about custody issues and legal outcomes in the lives of their therapist. In the 1960s, custody was usually awarded to the mother; only on rare occasions did fathers obtain custody. Not surprisingly, as therapists tend to be nurturing and concerned about the emotional development of children and are more aware of their own needs to parent, there was an increase in the frequency of custody issues in the male therapist group.

Patients expressed a need to understand the legal complexities involved in the divorce process and believed that the therapist should be knowledgeable and able to help them. If the therapist was able to encourage good communication and understanding with the attorney, the patients worked better in treatment. However, if through countertransference problems the therapist became competitive with the attorneys, treatment could be adversely affected.

Patients choosing their therapist from a small number of therapists caused another problem: the chance to meet a friend in the waiting room was greatly increased. Therapists were initially concerned about this but soon recognized that they were more concerned about it than were their patients. Most of the patients were temporarily made anxious by the possibility of this happening, but were able to continue the treatment relationship without difficulty.

Certain law offices had lawyers who specialized in divorce cases, and as a result there was the increased possibility that a therapist and a patient would meet in the law office waiting room, thus possibly violating patient confidentiality. The therapists, however, were more concerned about these chance meetings than were their patients. Attorneys accommodated their clients by carefully scheduling appointments to minimize the chance of such meetings. To avoid the problem, attorneys in two cases turned over their clients to a partner. This set up a transference-countertransference issue that centered on rivalry between patient and therapist, increased the patient's guilt, and underlined the stigma of being a patient.

The issue of secondary gain was an important concept. There tended to be a belief that women involved in divorce entered into psychiatric treatment to punish their husbands; it was costly, interminable, and their estranged husband would have to pay the bill. This, of course, was not generally the case. For example, a young mother asking for custody was more afraid that the stigma of mental illness would be held against her in the court process, thus outweighing any possible secondary gain. The secondary gain factor was increased in some patients when money, not custody, was the only quantifiable item.

Therapists reported complex and uncomfortable countertransference reactions when an estranged spouse was in treatment with another therapist. Their patients were generally aware of this, which tied in closely with their fantasies of the therapist-spousal relationship. Few patients perceived this situation initially in shades of gray: the black or white projection depended on the nature of the transference.

CONCLUSIONS

Supervision with a trusted colleague is especially important when the therapist's personal life is distressed, as it is during divorce. Grief can fog the therapist's thinking about patient issues, creating countertransferential blind spots. Therapists mourning a death usually return to clinical work before their grief work is complete, and those divorcing may interrupt work only for brief courtroom appearances. Reasons for this early return to work vary, but it results in therapists' attempting to help patients while still in pain themselves:

> Discussing cases with nonjudgmental supervisors helps therapists sharpen their clinical thinking and keep their own needs separate from those of their patients. Supervisors need to avoid shaming an already suffering therapist with their comments, which is easy to do with pointed statements like, "Watch your countertransference!" or, "You're really not seeing this clearly at all." Observations made more gently have a better chance of appropriate digestion and use by the therapist. Also, supervisors need to support therapists emotionally, which may include referral

for personal psychotherapy. Other professional colleagues can help by treating the divorcing therapist's loss as real and remaining empathic. Sometimes great relief may be gained from a colleague's permission to discuss this "socially unspeakable" loss. When such support is extended it becomes more likely that patients will be treated appropriately. (Pappas 1989, pp. 514–515)

Countertransference issues that develop in the course of therapy can aid or hinder treatment, depending on the nature of the reaction. In this chapter, I have looked at the special countertransference reactions that can arise between a therapist, his or her supervisor, and his or her patient when all three are involved in the divorce process.

The positive effects of supervision on countertransference need to be emphasized. There is a concern that supervision or concurrent treatment of the therapist could be invasive or deleterious to the primary patient-therapist dyad. In his discussion of how the parallel process of supervising a therapist (in the process of divorce) who is working with a patient (also in the process of divorce) can produce countertransference as a vehicle for understanding the patient, Weiler (1989) wrote, "Most countertransferences seen in supervision do not indicate pathology in the supervisee but are expectable and largely normal reactions to the patient's transference. When the supervisors share their countertransference reactions toward the patient with the supervisee . . . and foster comparison of countertransference reactions followed by cognitive elaboration, the experience of invasion of privacy should be rare. The 'parallel process' model can also be a vehicle for the supervisor to share personal reactions and thus clarify the 'rhythm of the dance' that the patient leads" (p. 290).

The theoretical stance taken in this discussion of countertransference issues is that the accurate analysis of countertransference will lead to a deeper understanding and that supervision can be helpful in the analysis by the described interaction to the therapist. It was the very fact that the therapists became aware that they were in the midst of a "transference-countertransference neurosis" that led them to seek help.

This is a retrospective review that raises questions that deserve further exploration. A prospective study would lead to clearer guidelines for therapists to either treat or refer the patient if the potential for nontherapeutic transference-countertransference reactions are present. It is clear in this study that the greatest risk was when the patient and the therapist were in phase II of the divorce process and stage III of loss. The second highest risk was when the patient had moved further along the continuum of resolution than had the therapist. The limitations of a retrospective study do not allow more in-depth analysis. The countertransference issues and reactions described here are not new, but the focus is.

The material presented came from a small group of patients, therapists, and supervisors who had one thing in common: they were all involved in various phases of divorce. This specific area was focused on in an attempt to increase awareness and understanding of the complex issues involved and to encourage more therapists to treat patients with a wide variety of problems in the various phases of separation and individuation by lessening their concern of encountering unworkable countertransference reactions. The common bond of their human condition can enhance the countertransference phenomenon and increase the effectiveness of treatment.

REFERENCES

Abend SM: Serious illness in the analyst: countertransference considerations. J Am Psychoanal Assoc 30:365–380, 1982

Abend SM: Countertransference, empathy, and the analytic ideal: the impact of life stresses on analytic capability. Psychoanal Q 55:563–575, 1986

Bellis JM: Countertransference: an odyssey. Paper presented at the Proceedings of the Pacific Northwest Conference on Bio-energetic Analysis, August 1989

Freud S: The future prospects of psycho-analytic therapy (1910), in The Standard Edition of the Complete Psychological Works of Sigmund Freud, Vol 11. Edited and translated by Strachey J. London, Hogarth Press, 1957, pp 141–151

Glaser RD, Borduin CM: Models of divorce therapy: an overview. Am J Psychother 40:233–242, 1986

Heimann P: On counter-transference. Int J Psychoanal 31:81–84, 1950

Heimann P: Counter-transference. Br J Med Psychol 33:9–15, 1960

Mann J: The management of countertransference in time limited psychotherapy: the role of the central issue. International Journal of Psychoanalytic Psychotherapy 10:205–214, 1984-1985

Norcross JC, Prochaska JO: Psychotherapist heal thyself, I: the psychological distress and self-change of psychologists, counselors, and laypersons. Psychotherapy 23:102–114, 1986

Pappas PA: Divorce and the psychotherapist. Am J Psychother 43:506–517, 1989

Weiler MA: Countertransference and supervision (letter). Am J Psychiatry 146:290–291, 1989

Chapter 7

Pregnancy: The Obvious and Evocative Real Event in a Therapist's Life

Maureen Sayres Van Niel, M.D.

A therapist's pregnancy affords one of the most influential of all "real" events in the therapeutic relationship. Because the pregnancy is obvious and its meaning evocative, a reaction to the situation is unavoidable. In this chapter, I examine the effects of such an event on the therapist, the patient, and the therapeutic relationship. My clinical observations of 12 patients in psychoanalytic psychotherapy and my own reactions to my two pregnancies over a period of several years are used to examine issues such as the nature and pattern of patients' transference reactions, the evolution of these reactions during different stages of pregnancy, the nature of one therapist's countertransference reactions, the decision about when or if to tell the patient, practice attrition, supervision of a pregnant therapist, and the impact of this "real" event on the therapeutic alliance and outcome of these therapies.

BACKGROUND

Early theoreticians paid little attention to the important event of a therapist's pregnancy, so our knowledge of this event and its effect on the psychotherapeutic process is limited to the findings of several authors who have written on the subject over the past three decades (Bassen 1988; Fuller 1987; Lax 1969; Nadelson et al. 1974).

To summarize what has been observed about a therapist's pregnancy we can begin in the 1950s, when Bibring (1959) described the psychological impact of pregnancy in general. She stated that "preg-

I wish to express appreciation for the review and suggestions on the content of the chapter by Roberta Apfel, Arthur Kravitz, Kathryn Kris, George Vaillant, and Arthur Valenstein.

125

nancy is a period of crisis ... leading to the revival and simultaneous emergence of unsettled conflicts from earlier developmental phases" (Bibring and Valenstein 1976, p. 359). She also noted, "Stress is inherent in all areas: in the endocrinologic changes, in the activation of unconscious psychological conflicts pertaining to the factors involved in pregnancy, and in the intrapsychic reorganization of becoming a mother" (Bribing 1959, p. 116).

More specifically, Bibring et al. (1961) described three emotional phases an expectant mother experiences. The first is characterized by an enhanced preoccupation by the woman with herself and her bodily changes. Then, with "quickening," the mother begins to see the baby as potentially separate from herself—that "the child will always remain part of herself, and at the same time will always have to remain an object that is part of the outside world and part of her sexual mate" (p. 22). Finally, a maturational integration occurs that allows the woman to add the role of mother to her identity. Bibring warned that the maturational integration resulting from a pregnancy is more gradual than had been previously expected.

In the late 1960s, Lax (1969) elaborated on Bibring's perceptions (1959) by specifically addressing the pregnant therapist: "Pregnancy in an analyst will stir up in the analyst some echoes of topical childhood conflagrations" (p. 363). Lax suggested that the pregnant therapist is therefore "more vulnerable than she would be otherwise to the different transference reactions of her patients" (p. 363). She also indicated that the neutrality of the therapeutic relationships is affected by the presence of a real event in the therapist's life. Among the common countertransference reactions she noted were that some therapists were "blind and deaf to veiled allusions related to their conditions" (p. 371), some experienced a noticeable amount of guilt, and some met the envy and greed that occurs for some patients with either excessive concern or anger.

Lax (1969) went on to say that for the patient, the experience of an analyst's pregnancy is unique in that it is a "highly charged stimulus and evokes deep-seated childhood conflicts, fantasies and wishes" (p. 363). Her patients commonly experienced intensified transference reactions with themes of rejection and loss, sibling rivalry, Oedipal conflicts, denial, anger, and envy. She emphasized the difference in her male and female patients' responses, noting the presence of stormy transference reactions to her pregnancy only in her female patients. Finally, she found that identification, taking various forms, was the most common defense employed by the patients, pointing out its ability to allow the patient "narcissistic gratification and compensation."

To the above, Paluszny and Poznanski (1971) added that unconscious stimuli often prompted pregnant therapists to initiate more discussions of children from the patients than usual. They also suggested that some withdrawal occurred for therapists in the second and third trimesters: "Hence, feelings of rejection by many of the patients had a reality basis" (p. 274).

After confirming some of the above findings, Benedek (1973) and Nadelson et al. (1974) addressed the complexity of reactions from coworkers to a therapist's pregnancy. Nadelson et al. (1974) also referred to the changes in the therapeutic process when a therapist's sexuality is so blatantly observable and a "third person" is in the room: "If a therapist remains aware of her changing perceptions, conflicts, and needs, she will be better able to hear her patients' concerns as they evolve during the pregnancy" (p. 1111). They also concluded that "most patients deal productively with conflicts as they arise in the context of pregnancy, and, in fact, working through these conflicts often provides a particularly effective therapeutic experience" (p. 1111).

Balsam and Balsam (1974) and Fuller (1987) observed that changes in the thoughts and behaviors of the therapist and patient during a pregnancy could be divided into different stages in relation to the pregnancy, according to the timing of their occurrence, including the pre- and postpartum period. Fuller also was the first to be specific about the important role a supervisor plays in support of the therapist during a pregnancy.

Finally, Bassen (1988) collated the opinions of 12 analysts who had had pregnancies. She concluded that "when it was possible to work through the intensification of transference and resistance stimulated by the pregnancy, the patients developed an enhanced sense of conviction about the power of denial and other defenses and the existence of unconscious wishes and fantasies. . . . For the analyst, it was often difficult to find the right balance between being appreciative of and tactful in response to patients' genuine caring and concern while dealing with their interest in the pregnancy and the baby analytically" (p. 283).

CLINICAL MATERIAL

Observations in this chapter are based on work done with all 12 patients I treated in psychoanalytic psychotherapy over the course of the several years surrounding my two pregnancies. The group is somewhat homogeneous in that there were 11 women and only 1 man, most were in their twenties to forties, most had neurotic and characterological disorders that had not required hospitalization, and all had been in treatment about the same number of years. (I had begun my practice about 3 years before my first pregnancy.) All of the patients were heterosexual, and all had siblings. Some were married, but most did not have children as yet. Notes were taken from early in the first pregnancy, during the second pregnancy (about 20 months later), and up until 4 years later.

Before discussing clinical material, it is important to state that the response of an individual patient or therapist to a pregnancy will, at one level, be unique and will represent a product of his or her own temperament, biological makeup, life history, parenting, and stage in treatment. Nevertheless, as a pregnant therapist, I did note interesting patterns in the responses of most of my patients.

First Trimester

Nine of the 12 patients did not mention the pregnancy for the first 3 to 5 months despite my more frequent schedule changes and obvious fatigue. At the time, even before consciously acknowledging my gravid state, patients had experiences of unconscious identification with me. Two of the patients ceased having menstrual periods in the fourth month of the pregnancy, having no medical basis for such, only to have them resume at the time my periods resumed postpartum. Four patients gained 20 pounds over the course of the pregnancy, and then lost them in the year following the delivery. In the eighth week of the pregnancy, one patient reported a confusing sensation of feeling sick only in the mornings, much "like a pregnancy," an impossibility in her life at the time.

During this time, my own denial took the form of not admitting the physical toll that early pregnancy was taking on me; I was denying the need to change my schedule to include more rest periods. The presence for me of denial and primitive associations was evident in an example on the one day that I was so nauseous I had to leave the room, saying as I left, "Excuse me, I will be right back. I have something caught in my throat."

Before the point that most patients acknowledged the pregnancy, I occupied myself with pragmatic questions as to how to manage the maternity leave, my bodily changes, amniocentesis, what to share with patients about the experience, and when to share it. When the patients eventually acknowledged the pregnancy, they also began asking me many pragmatic questions, such as "When is your due date?" "Are you having amniocentesis?" and "How long is the expected break in therapy?" I had difficulty negotiating the discussion of these matters, at times feeling compelled to answer questions about myself in a way that I had not felt previously.

Second Trimester

The point at which most patients acknowledged the pregnancy was the time when I was experiencing the very critical "quickening," had heard the fetal heart beat, and had seen the fetus on ultrasound. It was a time of great excitement and awareness of the reality of a new life within me.

As the patients learned of the pregnancy, competitive behaviors developed. One single woman furiously began proceedings to take in a foster child before she recognized the connection to the pregnancy. Another, a physician, talked about changing her career to obstetrics. The male patient demonstrated a period of exaggerated competition with colleagues and successfully competed for jobs that he had previously avoided for years.

Some patients acted out. One patient, a family planning expert, seriously jeopardized her intimate relationship by having unprotected sex with casual acquaintances. A direct interpretation was necessary for the patient to see the transference component in her actions; she was making an effort to "go out and get her own baby" in the face of the pregnancy.

Although these behaviors now seem obviously related to the pregnancy, as they developed I was often not able to see immediately how they related to it. Supervision and analytic treatment were extremely helpful in sorting out the patients' and my own complex reactions. For those patients who had not mentioned the pregnancy by the end of the second trimester, I brought up the matter for discussion.

Third Trimester

Appropriate interpretations of the patients' competitive and acting-out behaviors begot an important period of intensification of the maternal transference in most patients' treatment. This transferential reaction often took the form of a temporary regression, with increased passive longings, anger, and hostility.

On examination, these reactions were often duplicating some actual patterns in the patients' early mother-child relationship. Patients talked of new feelings of helplessness and "paralysis," yearning for my advice on almost every subject. They talked of "just wanting to be picked up and touched" or of feelings of emptiness in the face of me, "who is so full." One woman associated to the constricting feeling of being zippered into her crib covers as a young child crying to be let out.

A recrudescence of the disappointment that they did not have 100% of my, or anyone's, attention occurred for many of the patients at this time. A graduate student with an A average got Cs and Ds on several tests. An accomplished scientist became insecure about giving Grand Rounds because of anxiety and a lack of self-confidence. An entrepreneur demonstrated depressive and hostile moods that produced admonitions from her supervisor.

Negative transference in the form of hostility and sadism was demonstrated in patients at this time as they began to cope with the reality of the impending separation, their own competitiveness, and the real dangers associated with birth. They began associating to stories of fetal abnormalities and miscarriages that they or others had experienced, casually dismissing their intent or fears by saying "Of course, yours won't be like that!" One patient went through a period characterized by pouting, easy disappointment, and impertinence toward me, causing her to comment finally that she reminded herself of her friend's 13-year-old daughter. "Oh," she said, "That's how old I was when my brother was born. . . . Things were never the same for me after that."

Many patients were overly concerned that I was distracted, and "thinking about your baby," and they had an exaggerated fear of my losing interest in them after the birth. At different times during the pregnancy, many patients experienced a noticeably heightened sense of sexuality. Patients reported a new awareness of men and their "powers": the male patient reported a heightened awareness of his own sexuality and sexual drive, including an opening up of "animal-like sexual feelings." One female patient began experiencing the world as "ruled by testosterone," and two others became acutely hostile toward men, temporarily wishing not to associate with them.

The interpretation and observation that the patients' behaviors were similar to experiences in their own early relationships with their mothers led to an influx of new, early-life associations and memories that had often not been recalled previously in therapy.

Several patients had memories of their mothers' subsequent pregnancies, including scars and shorn bodies that their mothers had come home from the hospital with and their parents' joy at the arrival of their new siblings. One remembered the puzzle of a bus she did at age 3 that served as an entrance test to a New York private school. Another remembered merrily pounding the hammer of his toddler toy, trying to dislodge the pieces and attract his parents' attention. Another remembered long hours of her mother's coaxing and rewards during early toilet training. This more positive phase of transference was often accompanied by a series of memories of former surrogate mothers who had rarely come up during previous years of treatment. What emerged was the previously unreported amount of primary mothering that was actually done by nannies or grandmothers.

At the time of the maternity leave, the natural excitement and anxiety about the birth by both the patients and myself carried an element of joy from a separate world than the one we had previously shared in the treatment process. Besides having memories of their early lives, most patients mobilized more positive defenses, like humor, to reckon with my departure. As I waddled off to my maternity leave, one patient slyly stated that she was happy to have the experience of seeing "new dimensions" of me.

Immediate Postpartum Period

After a relatively uncomplicated delivery and a maternity leave of about 10 weeks, a new period of questions and fantasies began in which the patients explored and tested how far the boundaries extended in this new, more "real" relationship (the "presence" of the baby in the room before birth). At this time I found myself again feeling obligated to tell the patients something about the birth of the baby, the name, and the gender. I found it difficult to rapidly integrate the new role and reorganize my life as a therapist and a first-time mother, especially given that the patients really had been for some months unavoidably "part" of my more private life.

On the other hand, when I returned from leave, four patients commented that I seemed surprisingly undistracted and able to get "back to business" right away. One of these patients, in later discussing the pregnancy and its effect on her, said that my readiness to work forced her to see that it was she who had been "hoping for more of a vacation from my problems."

When the formalities of my return had been completed, there was an interesting period of associations on the part of the patients to babies—what they had meant to them, what they were like, what their siblings had been like, what it was like to care for siblings, and interesting dreams about babies. Several patients had dreams that I was their mother and their age in the dreams corresponded to the number of years that they had been in treatment with me (e.g., one patient had a series of dreams with me as her mother when she was 4 years old, the number of years she had been in therapy). Analyzing the patients' projections of babies' activities and interests gave insight into the patients' perceptions of themselves in relationship to me at that time.

Interestingly, the most difficult, affect-laden period relating to the pregnancy seemed to occur *after* the birth for most patients. About 9 months after my departure, a critical phase in the experience of my pregnancy occurred. It was at that time that most patients experienced the painful affects brought on by those memories recalled right before my maternity leave. These affects were those associated with the patient's early life, with preeminent themes of fears of abandonment, loneliness, sibling rivalry, and recognition of their separateness. Many entered a period, lasting about 6 months, of painful affect in relationship to their mothers. Commonly, the patients felt deep feelings of sadness, loneliness, and acute feelings of loss and separation, not knowing "how I will fill the void." One patient described it as a feeling of intense loneliness: "Like a hollow wind blowing across a Scottish moor." Another patient had recurrent nightmares of being left abandoned and helpless by her husband during a nuclear holocaust. Several patients who had especially pathologically fused relationships with their mothers suffered a great deal at this time, seeming finally, after months of painful affect, to be able to look critically at the symbiosis they had theretofore fantasized about before and during the pregnancy.

The patients who did not experience clearly discernible affects during or right after the pregnancy later had occasions when intense, inappropriate affects emerged in response to mundane situations. For example, one patient burst out crying while watching the evening news report about a particular presidential candidate. "The world is run by pygmies!" she declared in outrage, followed by an outpouring of sadness that lasted for hours and ushered in a new period in treatment about her disappointing relationship with a distant mother with five other children. Although she had been unable to confront her reaction directly, both to my pregnancy or to her mother, the affect continued and was eventually expressed directly. Overall, this was a period of growth and grief for patients over early disappointments with parents and required more involvement, patience, and bearing of painful affect by me.

Unfortunately, though, about this time I experienced difficulties. I found myself physically weary and impatient in response to the demands of the sad patients. In fact, their affects were the natural and intensified evolution of the therapeutic work and were appropriate. They were not acting out, but, feeling the intensity of the demands of my own child, I found their affects more burdensome than at other times.

For example, I detected my obvious weariness at one point when I found myself doing things I do not ordinarily do. I was so frustrated with the depressed patients that I actually began to make an appointment for one of them with an adjunctive therapeutic practitioner, a job counselor. Again with supervision, I realized that at that particular time I had unresolved dependency conflicts of my own, and with adequate support and more rest these feelings gradually subsided.

By about a year after the birth, the resolution of the grief and separation was occurring for most patients, and this resolution blended into the therapeutic work in progress before the pregnancy. The patients seemed to have achieved some integration of the event, making statements, such as "Well, I am not married yet as I hope to be. I have not yet got the child that I hope to have, but I have created something else of value; my composition has been chosen to be performed by the symphony this fall."

SECOND PREGNANCY

About 20 months after the birth of my first child, I became pregnant again. My practice had remained quite stable over the 2 years; I was still treating all but one of the same patients (one patient moved away), which afforded ready comparison. One of the first things I noticed was that 2 years in a child's life was obviously much longer than 2 years in a patient's life.

The second pregnancy loomed much less large than the first pregnancy had for both me and for the patients. The experience therefore got significantly less play in my own consciousness, and it was my perception that the absence of the newness or fears of the unknown made for much less fanfare in the room for both the patients and myself. I perceived that the clinical responses of the patients were similar but muted compared with those to the first pregnancy. In addition, I felt noticeably freer to explore and identify them when they did occur. I noticed much more readily that I was denying some of my own reactions or needs. For example, I realized that my own excessive nurturing energy and thirst during breast-feeding had led me to suddenly provide a water cooler with tea in my waiting room. I also realized this time around that my denial during the first pregnancy may have been more present than I had initially recognized.

During the second pregnancy I found myself at times more likely to introduce the anticipated maternity leave earlier. In March, I knew that I would be away much of August, September, and October, and so I brought it up at times where appropriate to facilitate patients' plans for vacations, trips to the Far East, or the like requiring advance planning. For these patients, I was not as concerned with "burdening the patient" with the information too soon, partly because the first pregnancy afforded a full exploration of their fantasies and associations and partly because of my own desire to "get on with it."

After delivery of my second child, I gained further insight into the patients' painful and symptomatic period 9 months after the maternity leave began. It did recur during this pregnancy for most patients, although with diminished intensity. Their "deterioration" seemed to correspond best to the time when I was emerging from the postpartum period and its inherently instinctual, demanding, and rewarding nature. It was about this time that I weaned the baby, took off my postpartum weight, went back to exercising, and felt more energy. The baby had been "launched" to a certain point, which made me more relaxed and self-centered and in some ways more receptive to the needs of the patients, who at that time seemed to increase their symptomatology. The timing of these patients' most intense reactions may have had to do with a conscious or unconscious effort on the part of the patient to protect me or not try to "get" from me what I could not tolerate at some level. With resolution of these affects and continuation of the treatment, the patients talked much more the second time about their own wishes or lack of wishes to become parents themselves.

Another important difference in my second pregnancy was that although it ended in a healthy outcome, it ended earlier than expected (at 35 weeks instead of 40 or 42, as it had during my first pregnancy). This created certain problems that are relevant to the many women for whom the final trimester does not go as planned and they are forced into bed rest or the like. Because I had preeclampsia requiring immediate induction of labor, I was surprised and worried about the outcome. Moreover, the anxiety of the patients when an appointment is abruptly canceled and no plans are made for rescheduling during a pregnancy was also obvious. To allay the fears of the patients without intruding terribly on my own privacy, I made brief calls to patients as soon as I was over my own worry and shock to tell them that both the baby and I were fine. The precipitous ending created difficulties for several patients that may not have occurred without that development.

I made no further contact with my patients during the maternity leave. Although I had had someone cover my practice during my first leave, during the second I took phone calls myself, leaving the option for actual visits with a covering physician. There were only four calls in the 3 months, which I did not find onerous.

A problematic approach was brought to my attention by one resident who relayed to me a poor outcome in her practice when she went into premature labor at 31 weeks and actually delivered a premature infant at that time. She "refused" to talk to or refer for help the patients who phoned her and felt extremely intruded on by them as they furiously sought answers to their fears about the welfare of her and the baby. She had felt so completely overwhelmed for several months that she did not make contact with the patients, who were extremely symptomatic, had hospitalizations, and sometimes left therapy.

It is impossible to keep the patients entirely out of the outcome of this process once it has been in the room and subject for discussion for 8 months. It would seem minimal for someone to call at some point after the delivery, with the news that mother and baby are fine if that is the case. I found it useful to ask the patient how they would like to be notified; some chose a note and others a phone call.

Because my interest in this subject became known, colleagues began sharing experiences of their own about the effect of pregnancy on their patients and on themselves. Several additional issues were raised. The first is that there seems to be a rumor circulating in the psychiatric community that you can plan to lose about one-third of your practice when you have a pregnancy, and indeed many women reported this was the case for them. For some patients, the experience was unbearable, no matter what the reaction of the therapist, and they left.

There also seems to be a countertransference issue that prevails and diminishes the size of the practice, either wittingly or unwittingly. Many women clinicians find that when they become pregnant and face family life, they wish to work fewer hours than they had been working. For those entirely in private practice, it may mean patients are told that they might be "best managed in a team approach" or are suddenly referred for psychoanalysis, and the like. As one woman therapist put it, "Before my pregnancy, I used to analyze the resistance when a patient wanted to prematurely stop his or her therapy or decrease the number of hours they came. Now I find myself just letting it go so that my schedule will be lighter after the baby is born." Because this message conforms to the patients' worst fears about the experience of pregnancy (i.e., that they will be banished, rejected, and unimportant once the baby comes), it is helpful to be mindful of the difficulties in paring hours from one's practice once one is engaged in longtime psychotherapy with patients.

A LOOK BACK

Now that 4 years have passed, my perspective on the pregnancy experiences is a more objective one. Over these years, there have been enormous changes in me as a person and, therefore, as a therapist. I have gained an understanding of children and an understanding of the strains of parenting. I now also have a substantial respect for the different temperaments that arrive on the earth, seemingly with very different programs built in. I am more likely to understand the parents' perspective in trying to manage a certain set of behaviors. I have become aware of the complex interrelationship between a person's intrinsic nature, their circumstances, the dynamics of their upbringing, and the intrinsic nature of those rearing them. I see stages and moods that come and go and have a firsthand look at child development. And finally, I am more aware of my own limitations, temperament, and strengths.

There has also been a significant shift in me as a therapist since the pregnancies began. I have become much more relaxed, confident, and more comfortable with the therapeutic and "real" relationships since having children. Compared with the incredibly complex, demanding, and primitive feelings evoked by the mother-child relationship, the doctor-patient relationship seemed easy. All of a sudden, I could see many more patients in a day without a break and felt less laden with their affects or expressions of dependency. I feel more able to notice when I am testy with patients because of the vicissitudes of life with two young children. This may have occurred to some degree over time in any case because I have obviously also gained in years of experience as a therapist.

My patients and I seem to have a different relationship as well. We had been through something together (twice) that had changed the relationship. When I asked them how they thought, in retrospect, that the pregnancies had changed their therapy, to a person they thought it had been both difficult and beneficial. They were utterly delighted to be in my real life to some extent, and they felt they knew me and trusted that the therapeutic alliance was not "all a front" now. They felt they had had a living laboratory of what my "real feelings" were like. They also felt it had precipitated crises in the treatment that were intensely painful at the time, but felt resolved by termination.

I did find it helpful to have the somewhat rigid structure of psychotherapy to lean on at times to help contain the loosening of the relationship that has had to occur. I still do not bring things up about the children, even though the patients try to evoke these discussions as a test of how far the real relationship may go. I decide, as I had always done, how to respond to a particular patient's question. I do not feel I owe it to them to discuss the children at all times, just because they were at one time involved "in the room." As a therapist, I do not think I can easily negotiate the frequent disclosure of the details of my real life without sacrificing neutrality and sometimes subjecting the patients to my moods, personal biases, neuroses, or drives. I have noted also that what progress I might have previously attributed to a period of growth after the maternity leave may have been part of the expected outcome of the psychotherapeutic process. Changes made after the maternity leave were often not as permanent as the finalizing changes that did occur closer to termination.

CONCLUSIONS

Two reverberating mother-child relationships that are commingled in the office of a pregnant therapist raise fascinating issues for the therapy. First, those witnessing the unfolding of a pregnancy, be they patient or therapist, are forced by the power of the event to relive certain early stages of psychological development. Second, depending on the degree of outstanding conflict or resolution of these earlier stages, the pair will be more or less symptomatic during the pregnancy. Last, the symptomatology created in the therapeutic relationship occurs not only at the time of the pregnancy, but also during the several years after the birth of the baby.

The evolving fetus first rekindles wishes and fantasies of a perfect union, reflecting itself into the dyadic relationship between patient and therapist. Themes of attachment and loss, fears of abandonment and rejection, and, eventually, a separation and individuation evolve.

The attachment and loss issues in both the therapist and the patient are highlighted by a series of interactive separations. For the patient, the first separation is the one from the therapist, at the time that she is departing for maternity leave. A second separation of grander scope occurs later, with the loss of the metaphorical, all-gratifying symbiosis one imagines occurring in the womb. Birth into a separate world seemed a saddening reality that left a vacuum for most of the patients. Identification with the therapist and a new understanding of their real, less mystified mother-child relationship then arm the patient with the "knowledge" of the caring and parenting they did receive both at home and in the therapeutic relationship so that healthy separation can occur.

A series of separations also occur for the therapist throughout the pregnancy and postpartum period that of necessity stir up the therapist's own early developmental issues. First, there is a reminder at "quickening" that she is separate from the developing fetus. Then, there is a separation from both the patients and the pregnant relationship with the fetus at the time of delivery. Finally, at the time of weaning or other subsequent periods of separation and/or individuation for the child, the mother may again feel an awakening of her own attachment and loss or dependency issues. Guilt because of leave taking or "divided loyalties" may cause the therapist to reveal too much, only to feel slightly "overexposed" at some later date. A supervisor and therapist-analyst can offer added attention to the newly stressed mother-to-be, ensure that the clinical material is adequately reviewed, and help the therapist identify when she may be denying some of her own wishes as a mother, all of which arose in the clinical material presented in this chapter.

The infant, vestiges of whom remain in the room long after his or her birth, also elicits Oedipal themes of competition for patients. At first, the competition is experienced as hostility or a wish to actually have or do away with what the therapist has; later, it takes the form of increased striving for achievement in work, wishes to become parents themselves, and an increased awareness of their own sexuality and capacity for intimacy.

The observations in this chapter elaborate on previous discussions of the presence of the "third party" in the room during a therapist's pregnancy (Bassen 1988; Lax 1969). Although there is a substantial real component to the patient's complaints about the distractedness and preoccupation of the pregnant therapist toward the patient, there was evidence in this material that, though this was true to an extent, it was experienced with inappropriate intensity by many of the patients. This may actually represent the patients' projections of their own experience of the intrusion and distraction caused by the "uninvited" baby.

Previous discussions of the impact of a "real event" in a therapist's life on the psychotherapeutic process have aptly focused on the timing, wisdom, and meaning of the disclosure or nondisclosure to a particular patient of news, such as the death of a therapist's family member or a life-threatening illness (Givelber and Simon 1981; also, see Chapters 2 and 3). Pregnancy is similar, on the one hand, in that the therapist still carefully explores the meaning that the event will have to a particular patient based on his or her earlier life experiences. On the other hand, pregnancy must be disclosed and therefore can serve as a valuable probe to explore the more general questions of the "real" relationship. There is real joy, real danger, and real sharing during a pregnancy obvious to both the patient and the therapist. The patients will have seen you vulnerable but surviving, awkward but available, mothering and working. In the face of a life event as obvious as a pregnancy, the desires of the therapist to preserve personal neutrality and an unfettered flow of associations and fantasies simply cannot always be maintained (Hannett 1946; Lax 1969).

In this chapter I have pointed out some of the complex issues created by the existence of this unavoidable "real relationship." Paradoxically, pregnancy creates not only experiences of increased closeness to a therapist because a real-life event is shared, but also a visual reminder of the limits of the relationship. In response to the event, all of the patients studied felt that being a part of a real event in their therapist's life had been a helpful experience that produced new levels of closeness. The patients' ability to witness the real reactions of the therapist can be a helpful demonstration of the vulnerability, happiness, and sorrow that are a part of the richness and inevitability of a full human life.

However, there is evidence that, at times, significant reactions do occur in the therapist that have distinct implications for the work of the therapy (Bassen 1988; Fuller 1987; Lax 1969; Nadelson et al. 1974). Although it may be natural for a woman therapist who is pregnant or a new mother to undergo "developmental crises," preoccupying her with new experiences and conflicts, this may take the focus away from the patient and disrupt neutrality at times. Protection from these difficulties is promoted by the presence of a therapist-analyst and supervisor. Even for an experienced therapist, supervision and therapy-analysis from outsiders are valuable because of the dyadic intensity elicited by a pregnancy.

Pregnancy in a therapist provides a microcosmic view of principles of child development and issues that are characteristic of the psychotherapeutic process in general. Further study of this interesting issue would help define questions raised here, such as whether the response of a particular patient is predictive of the outcome of their therapy or what the difference in reactions of male and female patients are to the event or to issues such as a tragic outcome of pregnancy.

A woman therapist often enters a pregnancy unaware of the rich and primitive ride on which she has just embarked, both as a person and as a therapist. Although the real relationship that develops has benefits in demonstrating real human reactions, this very humanness is at the same time distracting enough to interfere with the therapy at times. The hope is that with much attention to these complicated processes, the outcome will more often be an integrating, enriching one.

REFERENCES

Balsam RM, Balsam A: The pregnant therapist, in Becoming a Psychotherapist. Boston, MA, Little, Brown, 1974, pp 265–288

Bassen C: The impact of the analyst's pregnancy on the course of analysis. Psychoanalytic Inquiry 8:280–298, 1988

Benedek E: The fourth world of the pregnant therapist. J Am Med Wom Assoc 28:365–368, 1973

Bibring GL: Some considerations of the psychological process in pregnancy. Psychoanal Study Child 14:113–121, 1959

Bibring GL, Valenstein AF: Psychological aspects of pregnancy. Clin Obstet Gynecol 19:357–371, 1976

Bibring GL, Dwyer TF, Huntington DS: A study of the psychological processes in pregnancy and the earliest mother-child relationship. Psychoanal Study Child 16(9):9–24, 1961

Fuller RL: The impact of the therapist's pregnancy on the dynamics of the therapeutic process. J Am Acad Psychoanal 15:9–28, 1987

Givelber F, Simon B: A Death in the Life of a Therapist and Its Impact on the Therapy. Psychiatry 44(2):141–149, 1981

Hannett F: Transference reactions to an event in the life of the analyst. Psychoanal Rev 36:69–81, 1946

Lax RF: Some considerations about the transference and countertransference manifestations evoked by the analyst's pregnancy. Int J Psychoanal 50:363–372, 1969

Nadelson C, Notman M, Arons E, et al: The pregnant therapist. Am J Psychiatry 131:1107–1111, 1974

Paluszny M, Poznanski E: Reactions of patients during pregnancy of the psychotherapist. Child Psychiatry Hum Dev 1:266–275, 1971

Chapter 8

Effects of Malpractice
Suits on Physicians

Richard B. Ferrell, M.D.
Trevor R. P. Price, M.D.

*"Can it be that they will take me too? Who are these men?" thought Rostóv
scarcely believing his eyes. "Can they be French?" He looked at the
approaching Frenchmen, and though but a moment before he had been
galloping to get at them and hack them to pieces, their proximity now
seemed so awful that he could not believe his eyes. "Who are they? Why are
they running? Can they be coming at me? And why? To kill me? Me whom
everyone is so fond of?" He remembered his mother's love for him, and his
family's, and his friends', and the enemy's intention to kill him seemed
impossible.*

Leo Tolstoy, *War and Peace*

These words, written by Tolstoy
to describe the feelings of young Nicholas Rostóv during the Battle of
Schön Grabern in November 1805, poignantly describe emotions that
we and others who have been medical malpractice defendants have
felt. Here are the sense of assault and violation, the feelings of outrage
and fear. Most painfully, here is the narcissistic injury, the astonishing
wound to our understanding of ourselves as admirable, well-meaning
people. Circumstances differ, but when we were accused of malpractice, Rostóv's incredulous fear was ours.

As attending physicians on a busy medical center hospital psychiatry service, we had some awareness that in our work of caring for many
seriously ill patients we were at risk of being named in a malpractice

We wish to thank Harry Beskind, who conferred valuable clinical perspective; Melanie
Cash, who gave cogent and balanced editorial comment; and Lucy Deyerle and Cynthia
Hewitt, who provided unstinting assistance in manuscript preparation.

141

action, but this awareness had a detached quality. We believed that if we worked hard, practiced conscientiously, kept ourselves scientifically up to date, and, most importantly, were attentive to our patients' needs and kept their interests foremost in our minds, the chances of being named in a malpractice suit were vanishingly small. We believed that we practiced in this way to the best of our abilities. We would not have argued with the view that malpractice suits happen to doctors who are out of date, inept, or indifferent toward their patients. This false sense of security, heavily laced with denial, ended abruptly when we were named as codefendants in a malpractice suit.

For the next several years we worked and lived in the penumbral darkness that this suit created in our lives. Other malpractice defendants are familiar with this shadow. There were the usual lengthy periods of apparent inactivity that afforded plenty of time for smoldering doubt and meticulous, often painful scrutiny of ourselves and of our treatment of our patient, now plaintiff. There were periods of heightened activity and great anxiety involving depositions, reviews and opinions by expert witnesses, and conferences with lawyers and insurance company representatives. One could describe the whole experience as being like a 6-year-long toothache, characterized by a baseline of constant, low-grade, gnawing discomfort punctuated by acute paroxysms of lancinating pain.

At last came the inevitable trial, which we believed would be a chance for vindication and closure. The trial, which had loomed for so long as a threat to our sense of personal and professional integrity and competence, now confronted us with the immediate, stark reality of standing accused in a public court of law of having negligently injured another person.

Transforming this personal anguish into a chapter, progressing from our individual anger and fear to a more detached perspective from which others might take something useful, was not easy. We needed to learn about our colleagues' experiences through their writing and, most helpfully, through personal contact and conversation. We talked with seven other physicians who were willing to give us detailed, candid appraisals of their own emotional responses as malpractice defendants. This chapter was written by them as much as by us. Conversations with these physicians plus our own introspections do not constitute a large or random survey of physicians' attitudes regarding malpractice suits, but we were impressed with how similar many of their feelings were to our own, as well as with how each of them brought to our attention some aspect of this complex subject that had not yet occurred to us. Their stories and observations are the basis for the rest of our discussion.

LITERATURE REVIEW

After the precipitous rise in the number of medical malpractice suits in the 1970s came an abundance of writing on the subject. Most of this writing views the malpractice phenomenon from a broad or societal perspective, examining unusual or precedent-setting medical or legal aspects of a particular case, considering the malpractice insurance crisis or some other financial aspect of the problem, or advising doctors both in generalities and in specifics as to how they might avoid suits. Precious little has been written about the effects of suits on individual physicians. Most of what does exist is by Sara Charles and her colleagues (Charles and Kennedy 1985; Charles et al. 1984, 1985, 1987), who have written three articles and one book on the subject.

Like ourselves, Charles's interest in the subject was piqued by having been a defendant herself. Her book, *Defendant: A Psychiatrist on Trial for Medical Malpractice* (Charles and Kennedy 1985), written with her husband, Eugene Kennedy, is an eloquent and compelling account of her trial, followed by an insightful discussion of the effects of the malpractice crisis on doctors, patients, and society. In the course of her work, Charles found 51 physicians in the greater Chicago area who were willing to be interviewed about their experience as malpractice defendants. In an earlier report (Charles et al. 1984) involving a questionnaire survey of 154 physicians who had been defendants, she suggested the possibility of two predominant symptom clusters.

The first cluster consisted of dysphoric mood plus at least four additional symptoms often associated with major depression. The second cluster, likened to adjustment disorder, was characterized by a "change in mood, inner tension, frustration, irritability, insomnia, fatigue, and gastrointestinal symptoms or headache" (Charles et al. 1984, pp. 564–565). This symptom cluster was attributed to a physical and emotional response to the stress of the malpractice litigation.

OTHERS' EXPERIENCES AND OUTCOME TYPES

Because our sources include only nine physicians, including ourselves, it is risky to generalize. We do think, however, that we can identify some recurrent, pervasive themes and some emotional responses that sued physicians are likely to experience. Being mindful of the uniqueness of each person's story, we think that we can broadly characterize three general outcome types with regard to resolution of emotional distress and to the successful continuation of professional practice.

Outcome 1: Seemingly Unscathed— None the Worse for Wear

Physicians in the first category give the appearance that all is well, and for the most part it is. After their experience with the malpractice suit, they continue their medical work as before, seeing patients and, in their own view, not changing their method of practice.

They do not become practitioners of excessively "defensive medicine," though most have an increased awareness of the importance of careful documentation in the medical record. They maintain an open and altruistic approach to their patients. Although they may, from time to time, reflect on their malpractice experience and regard themselves as sadder but wiser, they do not dwell on it, and it does not often intrude into their personal or professional lives. Still, when invited to recall and reflect on their experience, most of these physicians have vivid and painful memories and can describe in surprising detail the major events of the malpractice action, even many years later.

Generally, they do not have lingering symptoms of emotional or physical distress and seem to have come through their experience as defendants without obvious evidence of permanent emotional injury or functional disability. Yet one senses that they have been changed in some subtle ways. It is as if their sense of trust in and ability to care for patients without circumspection and without reservation have been somehow compromised. One psychiatrist noted that, "Since my trial, I find myself responding internally to patients in a way that I don't like. Before, if a patient would tell me about suicidal feelings, intentions, or plans, I would respond by trying to establish some rapport or connection with the patient, if this did not already exist. Then, assessing the patient's intent and the potential lethality of the situation, I would take steps to prevent injury, and then recommend a treatment plan, as any good psychiatrist would do. Now I often find myself distracted by thoughts of self-protection. How vulnerable am I if this patient harms himself? When I am thinking this way, I am not the kind of doctor I want to be. I resent having to spend mental energy to keep these thoughts in perspective so that I can keep the patient's interest foremost in my mind. I think this is a direct result of my trial." This negative effect was familiar to all with whom we spoke.

Another physician who seemed to have succeeded in coming to terms with most of the negative emotions arising from his malpractice experience said, "It is as if your wife had slept with someone else. Even though you might still care for her very much, you could never have exactly the same amount of trust again. The relationship would be changed in such a way that it could never fully be repaired." Although he had only been sued by one patient during his many years of practice, this simile seemed to capture the nagging sense of guardedness and the haunting quality of vigilance he now experienced in his relationships with his patients, a change that greatly saddened him. The following case example illustrates Outcome 1:

Case 1

Dr. A was sued by the family of a patient who had committed suicide. She said that she thought "lawyers could come at you in one of two ways. Either they can say that you are a good doctor who has committed some act of negligence, or they can launch a personal attack on you, questioning your motives and your integrity and accusing you of being a bad person." Dr. A felt that this second description fit the plaintiff's lawyer in her case. She said that the lawyer implied that she had not liked the patient and that she had allowed her countertransferential feelings to compromise treatment.

Dr. A was on the witness stand for 2 days. The pretrial period of discovery and deposition lasted for 8 years. Dr. A's husband was a lawyer; he had helped her keep events in perspective. She also had discussed the case with her medical colleagues, who had been quite supportive. During the trial they would stop by her office to ask how she was doing. After the trial she wanted to discuss the case further with her colleagues, so she gave an informal educational presentation about malpractice, which was emotionally cathartic.

The period of greatest anxiety was just before the trial. Dr. A felt that she had not become depressed at any time during these 8 years. She thought that she was able to put the pending legal action out of her mind and continue her professional and personal life satisfactorily except during the trial itself, when the proceedings and the anxiety associated with them weighed most heavily on her.

In retrospect, Dr. A felt that she had integrated this experience well. She did not think that she had changed the way she practiced, except that she now paid better attention to documentation. She had decided during the course of the legal process that she would try not to become bitter, practice defensively, or otherwise change her way of practice, regardless of the outcome. It seemed important to her sense of professional integrity, competence, and self-esteem that she did not feel that she had erred in the treatment of this patient.

On one occasion in the midst of the trial Dr. A encountered the plaintiff's lawyer in a social situation. The lawyer spoke to her briefly, saying "not to take it personally," a phrase several other physicians in our own sample had heard in one context or another, often from the plaintiff's attorney. Dr. A was astounded, as were the others, that the lawyer could say this but felt constrained from expressing her true feelings of rage because the trial was not yet concluded. She expanded on this idea, saying that she thought lawyers were really quite remarkable for their ability to treat events like her trial as just another day's work when, for her, it was a life and death struggle. She believed that if more lawyers were defendants in malpractice suits, they might develop a better understanding of defendants' feelings.

Thus physicians in this first category appear to have survived the process without major long-term deleterious effects. It is estimated that only about 6% of suits filed actually go to trial. Of these, as many as 80% result in a defendant's verdict (Gutheil 1989). It is tempting to suggest that if one is vindicated by a favorable verdict, one has a better chance of making a good emotional recovery, but this is not known.

In Charles's survey (Charles et al. 1985), only 1.6% of sued respondents had experienced an adverse trial outcome. This figure suggests that malpractice suits are an ineffective way of identifying inept doctors. Of our nine defendants, two cases are still unresolved; none of the other seven had experienced an adverse trial verdict.

Dr. A spoke of a sense of utter powerlessness and helplessness. Several of our nine defendants expressed similar feelings when realizing that opposing lawyers, in the words of one doctor, "can do anything they want with you. They can say or do anything they want. They're playing by their own rules, and there is absolutely nothing you can do about it." This sense of exposure, vulnerability, and helplessness before a powerful adversary frightened and angered many defendants. Dr. A seems to have been helped by an absence of previous severe emotional trauma, by a sense of personal and professional strength and competence, by the support of a knowledgeable spouse, and by supportive colleagues. She felt that she came through her trial well, but was not sure how she would have managed had she lost the trial. She was not at all sure that she would be able to continue working in medicine should she be sued again, although she said she would try.

Outcome 2: Survival With a Price—
The Walking Wounded

We regard a second category of resolution as a mixed or intermediate category in which emotional recovery seems to have been largely successful, but in which significant compensatory changes in the physician's life or type of practice occurred. Examples of this would include changing from clinical to administrative work, to reduce exposure to the risk of malpractice; eliminating certain types of patients from a practice, such as suicidal, psychotic, borderline, or surgical patients; or assuming an excessively defensive style of practice. As long as such physicians are able to reduce the risk of malpractice by such changes, they seem able to cope with the continuing demands of their work, though in a different, and often truncated and less stressful, sphere than they had prepared for, sought, and found gratifying before the suit. The following case example illustrates Outcome 2:

Case 2

Dr. B was sued by a patient who developed a surgical complication. The case went to trial and Dr. B won. He thought that he had won because his lawyer was better than the plaintiff's lawyer and because the plaintiff's expert witness "was a buffoon." Compassion for his patients was an essential part of Dr. B's view of himself. Even during the heat of the trial, Dr. B had continued to feel empathy for his former patient. On one occasion, he told his lawyer that he felt sorry for the plaintiff and wished that she could receive some compensation for the bad outcome.

At other times, Dr. B experienced feelings more typical of those of our other defendants. He recalled feeling angry and as if he were being assaulted by the plaintiff and her lawyer. He was amazed that the lawyers seemed to have so little understanding of or concern for his emotions. In his opinion, they regarded his trial as one would regard a business matter, whereas he felt that his entire professional life and integrity were at stake.

Dr. B said that some obstetric colleagues who had been sued several times each had told him that they had gradually come to regard malpractice suits as "coming with the territory," that is, an expected, albeit unwelcome, cost of being in the practice of medicine. Dr. B said that he did not think he could ever develop such an attitude. He felt that the suit had been a stress on him professionally and also on his personal life and on his family. He once wrote to his lawyer, asking if the legal proceedings could be moved along more rapidly because he was aware of many occasions when he would be talking with a patient and would be thinking about his malpractice suit instead of about the patient's difficulties.

After his trial, Dr. B decided to stop doing surgery, while continuing an office practice. He said that the suit affected this decision, but that it was not the sole reason. Even before the trial he had experienced frustration with the considerable time demands of his surgical practice and had been aware of wanting to have more time with his family.

Dr. B did not think that his trial had caused him to practice in any overtly defensive way, such as ordering unnecessary laboratory tests; however, he recognized a subtle but disturbing change in his attitude toward his patients. He trusted them less without intending to do so; he had come to regard his patients as potential adversaries. This was especially true if the patient's condition was not improving. At such times, when the patient most needed Dr. B's full attention, Dr. B was discomforted by an awareness that he was considering possible legal consequences for himself instead of concentrating on the patient's difficulties. He did not like this change in himself but was not optimistic about overcoming it.

Dr. B said that he became more meticulous in documenting clinical information and more obsessive in his thinking about clinical problems, especially if a patient was not improving. He assumed that lawyers and medical bureaucrats would consider this to be a desirable result of his experience with a malpractice suit. They might argue that his malpractice experience had made him a better doctor, but he believed that what had really changed was his greater tendency to be "on guard" and to protect himself.

During his trial, Dr. B had considered getting entirely out of medicine. He had discussed this idea with his lawyer, who had dissuaded him, with the now familiar argument that malpractice suits were something to be expected in the course of practicing medicine and should not be taken personally.

Dr. B, like several other defendants, held his own lawyer in high regard. When he felt overwhelmed by the anxiety of his situation, he found some relief in mentally placing himself in his lawyer's hands, hoping that the man's skill would save him. At the end of our discussion, he said that he would mention something unusual for whatever it was worth. He said that since his trial, he sometimes thought of his lawyer when having sex with his wife. He referred to this in a whimsical fashion, saying, "Maybe I need psychoanalysis." More likely, this simply reflects the intensity of his emotional attachment and feelings of gratitude and indebtedness toward his lawyer, feelings also described by several other defendants.

Outcome 3: The Halt and the Lame—
Permanently Damaged Goods

In the third category are doctors who appear to have been most seriously and permanently injured by malpractice actions. This outcome type includes instances in which physicians retire early, leave medicine entirely for some other work, take nonclinical jobs, or continue practice with serious unresolved emotional or physical symptoms that impair them professionally and personally and that seem directly attributable to their experience as defendants. The course of these individuals' lives may be significantly, persistently, and negatively altered by this experience, often irrespective of whether or not the legal action was warranted and of its outcome. The following case example illustrates Outcome 3:

Case 3

Dr. C had been sued on two occasions. Neither case went to trial. In the first instance, Dr. C was accused of having accepted a patient for hospitalization with commitment papers in which the petitioning physician had not filled out the form correctly. There was no allegation that Dr. C's treatment of the patient was negligent in any way. Dr. C felt sure that he had done nothing wrong and that he had helped the patient considerably. The suit was brought by a group of activist lawyers who were attempting to change the state involuntary hospitalization law. Malpractice suits were one means of bringing their concerns about the existing law to public attention. The malpractice suit against Dr. C was eventually dropped. He felt that he came through this experience quite well, due to his secure belief that he had not made a mistake and was therefore in a strong and defensible position. His awareness of the political overtones of the action was also very helpful.

The second suit occurred a number of years later. This suit was far more traumatic for Dr. C, perhaps because he had been sensitized by the first experience and also because, in this instance, he felt there was absolutely no ulterior motive that could explain the suit. This time, there was an allegation of improper diagnosis and treatment, despite the fact that Dr. C's involvement consisted only of signing an order while covering for a colleague. The particular order had no bearing on the patient's diagnosis or course of treatment, and Dr. C had never been involved in making a diagnosis or treating this patient. He was included in the suit only because he was one of several physicians whose names appeared in the medical record. Dr. C experienced this suit as capriciously unfair. He felt victimized and assaulted and eventually began to experience depressive symptoms with growing feelings of hopelessness and suicidal thoughts. He was continually preoccupied with the suit and with overwhelming anger and rage, particularly directed toward the plaintiff's attorney. He was unable to concentrate on his work and eventually sought psychiatric treatment himself.

About a year after the suit was filed, he became aware of an increasing preoccupation with memories of traumatic combat experiences in the Korean War. Nightmares about these experiences began to compound his difficulty with insomnia and fatigue. Dr. C eventually retired from medical practice and considered his retirement to be largely a result of this second suit. He later resumed part-time consultation.

The suit itself was eventually settled for a token sum without a trial. This outcome provided Dr. C with little relief. He continued to harbor feelings of intense anger and a fear of future vulnerability. If he received an envelope in the mail whose appearance held any hint that it might have come from a law firm, he experienced intense anxiety. Some aspects of this case suggest a type of posttraumatic stress disorder.

Dr. C had entered medical practice as a young man out of a deep sense of altruism. His experience with malpractice suits had left him with feelings of embittered betrayal. He said that he felt sorry for young physicians who were starting out, wanting to help patients and wanting to do right for people, because they did not know what they were getting into. He said that he had tried to be conscientious and to help others whenever he could and that, in return, he had been injured for his efforts. He felt that, no matter how hard he might try or how much good he might do for others, he would always be vulnerable and could be faced with a suit at any time. He described the feeling of being sued "as though someone were to sneak up behind you and hit you in the back with an axe." Sometimes Dr. C fantasized that he would go to the office of the lawyer who had sued him and confront this man and ask him why he had done such a horrible thing, but he never did so. He wished that his experience could somehow be used to help others, so that he could see some justification for what had happened. (Now he feels that it was simply an unwarranted attack that left him with emotional injuries from which he had not yet recovered.)

DISCUSSION

In our discussions with defendants, some dominant ideas emerged. First was the feeling of injury, of vulnerability, and of a deep narcissistic wound inflicted by the malpractice action, a feeling of "Why should this be happening to me when I've tried to do so well, when I have tried to help people?" There is an affront to the doctor's essential view of himself as a good person, called into question by an allegation of negligence or stupidity; implicit is the assumption that if one were a really good doctor (person) this would not have happened.

Thus the accusation of malpractice becomes a source of shame and narcissistic injury. Morrison (1983, 1989) defined the ego ideal as "the set of goals, values, and esteemed objects toward which the ego strives." The ideal self, a closely related idea, represents "the subjective sense of how closely one approximates" the ego ideal. Shame and related affective states such as humiliation, apathy, and diminished self-esteem result when one regards the self as defective, incompetent, weak, flawed, foolish, or inferior. In short, one feels shame when one falls short of internalized standards.

Shame leads to concealment and withdrawal and evokes fear of abandonment and rejection. Several defendants spoke of wishing to hide from friends or colleagues or of a wish to leave medicine entirely. Whereas some spoke of the support of colleagues, others sensed vulnerability to perceived aggressive competitiveness in their medical peers. Furthermore, some defendants were advised by their lawyers not to discuss the case with anyone.

One doctor spoke of his medical colleagues in these terms: "Doctors are like everyone else. If you are accused of malpractice, people assume that there must be some reason, that you must have done something wrong. Also, if you admit how depressed you are, they may consider you to be an 'impaired physician.'"

Vulnerability of the ego with regard to an assault on the ideal self does not necessarily represent psychopathology. Those with less narcissistic resilience are at greater risk, but the enormity of the perceived failure often contained in the accusation of medical malpractice threatens even the relatively healthy person. We do suggest that the narcissistic vulnerability of doctors is enhanced by their tendency to have high standards for themselves. They rely heavily on medical competence and often on a sense of uniqueness or specialness in regulating their self-esteem. Seen from this perspective, a malpractice suit is a heavy blow. This kind of injury results from the accusation of failure and, as a psychological issue, is separate from the legal question of whether or not medical negligence actually occurred. The psychological remedy is self-acceptance, including of one's shortcomings, but this is not always easy. In some instances, psychotherapy may be needed.

The interests of the principals in a malpractice suit or trial are different. The plaintiff regards himself or herself as injured and deserving of compensation. The judge and jury members are interested in administering justice and doing their jobs well, as are the respective lawyers who wish to represent their clients well and win the case. The doctor-defendant is concerned with emotional self-preservation. The uniqueness of this position could explain the loneliness and fear of loss of control that defendants report.

The second idea that engenders great anger and fear is the feeling of loss of control: that the facts of the matter are not nearly as important as the skill of the lawyers or the skill and persuasiveness of the respective expert witnesses. In Dr. B's case, as in most cases, he did not pick his lawyer. The lawyer was picked by the insurance company. Dr. B felt lucky that his lawyer seemed better than the plaintiff's lawyer, but even this was something completely beyond his control and could easily have been otherwise. It could have been his expert who appeared foolish or ignorant on the witness stand or antagonized the jury with disastrous results for him, without the facts of the case having been any different than they were. These vagaries lead doctors to feel vulnerable and to wonder why they expose themselves to the risk of malpractice suits. We think it is this fear and feeling of vulnerability that lead physicians to retire early, change their practice, consider quitting medicine, or practice in a way that is more guarded or adversarial with respect to their patients than was the case before they were sued. Aside from the personal anguish suffered by the physicians, this introduction of an adversarial way of thinking into the practice of medicine has serious negative effects on both doctors and patients. The rules and adversarial nature of the legal system are thus injected into the relationship between doctors and patients, with unfortunate consequences for both.

Other defendants who have been through a trial have also commented on their surprise at discovering the crucial importance of a defense attorney who is "better" than the plaintiff's attorney and of expert witnesses who are "better" than the plaintiff's experts. "Better" witnesses are more credible, better prepared, more personally appealing or less obnoxious, more convincing, and more skillful and practiced at testifying in court. All the defendants have observed that the courtroom proceedings seem less like a quest for truth and justice than a high-stakes contest between opposing lawyers and experts. The defendant becomes incidental, assuming an unaccustomed passive role in the wings with the attorneys occupying center stage. This sense of passivity and helplessness in the face of a powerful opponent is common. Even as our culture has idealized physicians and the medical profession, likewise has it idealized judges, lawyers, and the judicial system. We expect and hope that the courtroom will be a place where disagreements are dispassionately aired and weighed and decisions based on fairness, correctness, and justice will emerge. This idealized expectation runs afoul of reality when the outcome of the process itself seems so heavily reliant on the skill and verbal dexterity of the opposing lawyers with their supporting casts of expert witnesses.

Yet another shade of emotional response emerged in discussions with one doctor. He felt that he had gone well beyond the call of duty, helping his patient avoid a life of institutionalization. He felt that his motives and his effort were exemplary; to him a lawsuit seemed utterly offensive and unfair. He was left with a great deal of anger and a sense of futility: "No matter what I do, even if I do something better than anybody else would have done it, they can still attack me without warning or justification, and there's nothing I can do about it."

It is worth noting that although medical school and medical training and medical practice are highly competitive, they are not openly adversarial. Doctors are unfamiliar and ill at ease with a system that is fundamentally adversarial, in which one is rewarded for successfully attacking someone else, be it the opposing lawyer or the opposing plaintiff or defendant. Doctors are used to decisions being made through a consensus approach. They seek areas of agreement, not clever destruction of another's arguments. Doctors experience such disagreements and attacks as highly personal, offensive, and rude or slanderous, whereas many lawyers seem to regard them as part of a day's work.

One defendant described arriving at the courthouse for the first day of his trial and seeing two television trucks in front of the courthouse. He asked the bailiff if they were there for his trial; he was told that the publicity was for a murder trial that was just concluding. This imagined notoriety was connected with a fear of public exposure and humiliation and with doctors' view of an allegation of medical malpractice as tantamount to being accused of a serious crime. The seriousness and moral weight of an allegation of medical negligence often become magnified in the mind of the physician.

Different defendants have found their own lawyers to be more or less helpful. Those who have gone to trial seem to have felt confident about their lawyers and felt that they were of great help. In one instance in which a suit was filed in a jurisdiction where the doctor no longer lived, the lawyer seemed remote and ineffective. One defendant felt his case was being handled by someone quite junior in a law firm and that, although he regarded the suit as a serious matter, the lawyer seemed to dismiss it as something not to be taken too seriously. This might be analogous to a medical situation in which a patient comes to an unseasoned doctor with a complaint of severe pain and the doctor dismisses the complaint as not being serious, without understanding or responding to the degree of discomfort and fear the symptom is causing.

A tenth physician informed us of a situation in which an ethics complaint was filed against her. After a protracted and agonizing series of hearings, she was exonerated. Her emotional distress was much like that of our malpractice defendants. A difference is that the allegation was not medical negligence, but ethical wrongdoing, if anything a more serious accusation. The case involved an evaluation she had made of children who allegedly had been sexually abused and who were involved in a custody dispute. The ethical complaint was filed by one of the parents. She remarked, "Looking back on the experience, I think that one of the most frightening consequences of such action is that people may back away from . . . giving opinions in situations which clearly cry out for . . . professional leadership. I do worry that we will all become avoiders and withdrawers, rather than leaders and givers of opinions."

We are aware of some instances in which a malpractice suit served to make easier a practice decision that was psychologically difficult. A physician who has harbored a wish to restrict practice, change type of work, or retire early may discover that a malpractice suit, like an illness, gives permission for the change.

As indicated by our sample of nine physicians, the subjective experience of being involved in a malpractice action and the effects of this experience on the individual's emotional and professional life are varied. They range from minimal, with little apparent impact (Outcome 1), to devastating, with profound disruption of the individual's life in general and diminished capacity to function as a physician in particular (Outcome 3). The information gleaned from our sample suggests these three broad categories of outcome, yet it provides little insight into why physicians going through a similar type of legal action should be affected so differently. We suspect that temperament, psychodynamic factors, a host of interpersonal and psychosocial variables, the individual's home and work environment, and aspects of the legal proceedings all combine to determine the result.

Which of these factors are critically important, and in what ways, is not yet understood. Age, sex, marital status, family stability, the extent and quality of social supports available during the legal action, the medical specialty of the sued physician, and his or her prior knowledge of and familiarity with malpractice may be important. Other variables include the type and severity of the plaintiff's injury; the duration of the suit and its final outcome; whether there is a jury verdict, adverse or not, or a settlement; and the size of the settlement or award.

SPECIAL PROBLEMS IN PSYCHIATRY

The specialty of the physician can itself be a significant variable in determining the effect of litigation. Psychiatrists have special vulnerabilities because of the importance of the doctor-patient relationship in treatment. Although the nature of the psychiatrist-patient relationship is similar to the doctor-patient relationship in other areas of medicine, the central role of the therapeutic relationship is a difference. There are two special aspects of psychiatric practice that merit our attention because of the problems they present as a result of the threat of malpractice litigation.

In psychiatry, and sometimes in neurology and neurosurgery, the physician must stretch the patient-doctor relationship in a paternalistic direction in order to practice ethically. The problem of paternalism in psychiatry has been cogently discussed by Culver and Gert (1982). In some neuropsychiatric illnesses, the central nervous system, the organ system that underlies judgment, is ill. Schizophrenia, mania, depression, and dementias in their most severe forms provide examples in which psychosis or cognitive dysfunction may impair judgment to a dangerous degree. In such instances, the psychiatrist may have to act against the expressed wishes of the patient to try to prevent even greater harm. In other words, paternalistic actions such as bringing about involuntary hospitalization or treatment or recommending guardianship are morally justifiable only when their aim is to prevent even greater harm such as serious injury or death. Such work is usually difficult enough; the overhanging threat of malpractice litigation raises the ante and requires even greater courage of those making such important decisions.

A second area of special vulnerability concerns psychotherapy and the importance of countertransference fear and anger. The skillful psychotherapist's art and practice depend on trust. Psychotherapy is essentially collaborative. It requires a fundamental confidence in the constancy and benevolence of the therapy relationship. The therapist must feel free to practice with a sense of creativity, to speculate, and to interpret without fear, or else the quality of the therapy suffers.

Several of the psychiatrists with whom we spoke, including some who have not been sued, spoke of the negative effect of the fear of malpractice suits on their psychotherapeutic work. A psychiatrist told us of her experience with a patient who sued her after inflicting serious self-injury. The patient claimed that the therapist should have prevented this suicidal behavior. The patient could be regarded as having a character disorder with borderline features. She entered treatment seeking help with feelings of anger and betrayal and injured herself when she believed that the therapist had let her down.

The therapist recognized many feelings within herself after the suit was filed, including sadness, anger, and dismay. Only much later was she aware of the importance of anger in the countertransference in the treatment of another patient. This patient frequently made long phone calls to the doctor late in the evening. In spite of her fatigue at these times and the unproductiveness of these calls, the psychiatrist felt constrained from confronting the patient about the calls. She realized that she was afraid that this patient might also harm herself and then sue. This fear exerted a controlling effect on the doctor with resulting anger. Eventually the doctor became aware how angry she was at this patient and then recognized several similarities in the personalities of the two patients. She became aware that her responses to this patient resulted from a mixture of genuine concern and apprehension that she might be sued again if she did not meet the patient's demands. We think that countertransference anger and fear may be especially significant clinical problems for psychiatrists who have been sued.

RECOMMENDATIONS

More study is needed so that understanding, support, and intervention can increase the proportion of outcomes in the first category. Even then, we believe that the long-term emotional consequences for physicians involved in malpractice suits are more permanent and harmful than has been heretofore understood, regardless of the outcome.

For example, in our sample of nine physicians, two who were in the Outcome 1 group experienced the conclusion of long-term marriages within 3 years after the end of their suit. We are not suggesting a causal relationship between malpractice suits and divorce, but we do think that the stresses of litigation on physicians and their families are profound and may potentiate the emergence of marital difficulties. Also, we are aware of two other instances in which lawyers advised their physician-clients to consider divorce as a way of protecting assets.

We believe that the malpractice experience changes physicians in significant and often undesirable ways. These changes compromise their ability to function in their accustomed professional roles. Whether or not such changes are preventable or reversible through group or individual psychotherapy is unknown. Also unknown is the effectiveness of adjunctive drug treatment aimed at mild or subclinical depressive or posttraumatic stress disorder symptoms. Whether such therapeutic interventions might make a difference is clearly worth investigating, given the human and professional costs involved.

How can physicians involved in a malpractice suit limit its effects on themselves, their families, and their practices? First, we believe, they can help prepare their own defense, cooperate with their lawyer, and serve as their own "in-house expert witness." Doing literature searches, educating their attorneys in technical matters related to the case, and providing ongoing consultation, are adaptive ways to cope with dysphoria, depression, anxiety, and a sense of helplessness. Also, like a good-hitting pitcher, the actively involved defendant physician can thus improve the chances of winning.

Second, recognizing the enormity of the stress, they can seek support from their attorney, spouse, family, friends, or colleagues. Sometimes, given this special type of violation, there may be a need for psychiatric help or, in some cases, for marital or family help. A strong, stable marriage or a loving family may provide an anchor, a "port in the storm," for some sued physicians. On the other hand, the severe and continuing sting of a malpractice action may threaten a shaky marriage or increase trouble in an already distressed family.

Defendant physicians tend to be reluctant to speak frankly about their experience to other doctors, especially those who have not been sued. They may talk angrily about malpractice as a political or social issue and rail about plaintiffs' attorneys, but this is not likely to be as helpful as is reasoned communication of knowledge and experience among colleagues. Forewarned is forearmed; a discussion of the process and its legal, personal, professional, and family implications can reduce the fear of the unknown and give some reassurance that this experience can be survived.

On a societal level, we believe that physicians should advocate for the passage of no-fault statutes and tort reform. We are concerned about the financial consequences of the present system relative to rising health care costs. Moreover, we decry the personal emotional cost to physicians and the resultant diminution of their capacity for humane openness and empathic care of patients.

One of our group of nine doctors worked on behalf of tort reform legislation in his state legislature and state medical society after his trial. Halleck (1983), who also wrote from personal experience, affirmed the protective effects of sublimation and social support. He also mentioned the therapeutic effect of physical fitness and exercise, an opinion with which we agree.

Measures can be taken to reduce the chance of a malpractice suit. Gutheil (1989) noted that it is important for doctors to educate their patients and to talk with them freely about possible results of treatment. In obtaining truly informed consent for any treatment or procedure, it is important for physicians to emphasize the real possibility of a bad or less than ideal outcome and to provide some estimate of its statistical likelihood. If untoward events do occur, physicians should assure their patients that they are concerned, care about them, and will not abandon them.

The doctor should care for the patient in the very best tradition of "being a doctor." This in the final analysis will always be the best means of dealing with the threat of being sued for malpractice. Robert Frost (1949) suggested that we "Choose Something Like a Star"—a higher perspective from which to view the human condition:

> So when at times the mob is swayed
> To carry praise or blame too far,
> We may choose something like a star
> To stay our minds on and be staid.

We must have compassion for those who are ill and have a means of compensating those who are injured by medical accident or negligence without yielding to an urge to blame and prosecute those who have tried to serve well.

REFERENCES

Charles SC, Kennedy E: Defendant: A Psychiatrist on Trial for Medical Malpractice. New York, Free Press, 1985

Charles SC, Wilbert JR, Kennedy EC: Physicians' self-reports of reactions to malpractice litigation. Am J Psychiatry 141:563–565, 1984

Charles SC, Wilbert JR, Franke KJ: Sued and nonsued physicians' self-reported reactions to malpractice litigation. Am J Psychiatry 142:437–440, 1985

Charles SC, Warnecke RB, Wilbert JR, et al: Sued and nonsued physicians. Psychosomatics 28:462–468, 1987

Culver CM, Gert B: Philosophy in Medicine. New York, Oxford University Press, 1982

Frost R: Choose Something Like a Star, in Complete Poems of Robert Frost. New York, Henry Holt, 1949, p 575

Gutheil T: Malpractice in psychiatry and the psychology of litigation: interview. Currents in Affective Illness 8(8):5–14, 1989

Halleck SL: Malpractice in psychiatry. Psychiatr Clin North Am 6:567–583, 1983

Morrison AP: Shame, ideal self, and narcissism. Contemporary Psychoanalysis 19:295–318, 1983

Morrison AP: Shame: The Underside of Narcissism. Hillsdale, NJ, Analytic Press, 1989

Tolstoy L: War and Peace (1869). Edited by Gibian G. Translated by Maude L, Maude A. New York, WW Norton, 1966, p 201

Chapter 9

Countertransference Reactions to a Patient's Sexual Encounter With a Previous Therapist

Malkah T. Notman, M.D.

Sex between a therapist and patient is not a new problem but has emerged into the public eye more sharply in the last few years. There have also been increased awareness of incest and sexual abuse in the family, more open attention to victims of rape and abuse in other settings, and some decrease in the condemnation of the victim. The rise in consumerism has contributed to criticism of and challenge to relationships that were previously more protected and to greater awareness of sexual exploitation in many power relationships. In this regard, the therapist is in a particularly sensitive relationship to a patient, as the transference that is important in achieving a therapeutic result also makes the patient vulnerable to its manipulation and to emotional and sexual exploitation. This can be a matter of degree and quite subtle.

Most therapists will encounter one or more patients who have had a sexual relationship with a former therapist. Sometimes this is the presenting problem, sometimes it emerges in the course of therapy, and sometimes it is a matter of rumor or hearsay. The therapist's reactions are due to many influences: they reflect social norms, the therapist's attitudes toward women and their sexual roles, attitudes about sex, and conscious and unconscious residues of the therapist's own personal history, fantasies, values, and relationships. They may be contradictory and conflicted. Anger and outrage may coexist with curiosity, even voyeurism. Some therapists may identify with the other therapist and some with the patient. Some feel as if this is a remote and unlikely possibility for them. In this chapter, I address the predominant countertransference reactions to a patient's sexual encounter with a previous therapist and the therapeutic issues in treating a patient with such a history.

Therapists' reactions can be considered under the broad designation of countertransference. The term *countertransference* has acquired a broader meaning than it had in the past. Originally it referred to a therapist's unresolved responses to the patient and to the patient's transference. It was implied that these responses were distortions and represented neurotic issues. Currently, the term is used to mean the therapist's total response to the patient, conscious as well as unconscious, and does not imply that these are necessarily distortions.

Attitudes about all aspects of sexuality have changed in the past two decades. There has been a greater openness about sexual behavior and experiences in the media, in literature, and in education. There has been a rash of popular books on how to enjoy sex more. There is more tolerance of extramarital sexuality. In the 1970s and 1980s, the speciality of sexual counseling brought sexual dysfunction into respectability as a treatable disturbance. Homosexuality is less hidden. Reporting of rape, incest, and sexual abuse has increased. Although it is unclear whether sexual abuse and rape have increased, it is generally acknowledged that behaviors that existed for a long time have been more frequently reported. There has been a similar shift in regard to patient-therapist sexual relationships. Events that sometimes occurred many years earlier have been reported and malpractice suits have been brought and won. As publicity has grown, patients who were too frightened or embarrassed previously have become willing to report their experiences. The long interval between the events and the reporting has in many cases not diminished the feelings of distress or the sense of violation and trauma. As is common with other traumatic sexual experiences, such as rape, the effects of patient-therapist sexual relationships are long lasting.

Professional ethics guidelines have been clear in the last decade in prohibiting sex between patient and therapist during therapy and after. These ethical guidelines existed in the past but were not taught explicitly nor widely discussed. Most professional groups currently do not regard the transference as resolved at the conclusion of therapy and therefore do not hold that a sexual relationship with a former patient is free of the potential influence of transference interfering with freely given consent.

There has been growing attention to these problems. Public and professional attitudes about sex between patients and therapists began to change in the 1970s when the mental health professions clearly stated that this behavior was unethical. Brodsky (1989) traced the recent history of this development. Although clinical and anecdotal data were abundant earlier, survey data were collected in the 1950s and 1960s but not publicly presented until the 1970s and 1980s.

Even though it was unacceptable officially, sex between patient and therapist was not rare. It was, however, rarely reported, and professional organizations did not act consistently. The damaging effects on patients were not universally recognized. It was probably a result of many influences that this began to change: the broad changes in society, the growth of the women's movement, attention to rape and other forms of victimization, and the increased presence of women as therapists in psychiatry and psychology, as well as in social work where they had always been predominant. Large awards for malpractice suits because of patient-therapist sex became public in the early 1970s. Professionals and organizations conducted further surveys of their members' practices (American Psychological Association 1975; Holroyd and Brodsky 1977; Kardener et al. 1973; Perry 1976; Pope et al. 1979).

In the 1980s a number of these surveys confirmed the general figures that were obtained as to the prevalence of this behavior (Bouhoutsos et al. 1983; Gartrell et al. 1986). In responses to self-reported questionnaires, about 6%–7.5% of male therapists and 1% of female therapists said they had had sexual involvement with patients. This prevalence seems similar for psychiatry and psychology and lower in social work (Gabbard 1989). Similar patterns probably exist in all fiduciary relationships involving men in positions of authority and women as patients or clients, such as in the clergy and law. The preponderance of the male-therapist–female-patient dyad is a consistent finding. This is also reflected in the percentages of ethics complaints in professional societies. There are some reports of male-male and female-female relationships and there may be more female-therapist–male-patient reports with the increase in women in psychiatry, but the overwhelming majority are male-therapist–female-patient relationships.

An anecdote told by one psychiatrist recalling his residency illustrates the changes in professional attitudes. He had been treating a difficult patient who made many demands. She frightened him with the threat that if he did not accede to a particular set of demands, she would broadcast that they had been having sex. The young psychiatrist was terrified. He asked his supervisor what he should do if the patient carried out her threat. The supervisor laughed and said, "Don't worry. If it gets out, patients will beat a path to your door." A sexual relationship was thus presented as an attraction. This would not be said openly today.

ATTITUDES OF THE PROFESSION

Sexual relationships between patients and therapists were known and, whatever private attitudes existed, were tolerated by the profession in the past. Marriages occurred, occasionally with disastrous outcomes (such as when a rejected former wife committed suicide), but in some cases, marriage seemed to legitimize the relationship. Jung was known to have had sexual liaisons with patients, as did other prominent psychiatrists who were chairmen of departments and leaders in the field. Intimate relationships with supervisees and students were also well known. Public discussion of any of these problems was considered "too hot," even when recognized to be detrimental to the patient.

A colleague who tried to discuss what he or she had heard from a patient would often not be believed and would have trouble finding support for taking action against the therapist, even if his behavior seemed grossly exploitative. One woman therapist described her dilemma when she was first referred a severely chronically depressed woman with a history of several unsuccessful previous therapies. She learned from the referring therapist that the previous therapist, who had administered several courses of electroconvulsive therapy (ECT), had had intercourse with the patient while she was in the confused postictal recovery phase. At first the patient was indeed confused as to what was happening to her, but then became aware of it and told her family. She changed therapists and, although she also told her new therapist, he took no action. The abusing therapist's behavior was well known in the community, but he was never prosecuted for it. All who were involved felt reluctant to initiate action or thought it would be ineffective, as it might have been.

Today, the pendulum has swung the other way, toward a much more punitive attitude in some instances. Nevertheless, many people are still reluctant to believe a patient's story about her sexual experience with a therapist, and the tendency to think the therapist's behavior is provoked by the patient is widespread. Patients are readily labeled as borderline or hysterical with the implication that the provocation follows from the pathology and sometimes the further implication that the patient then becomes responsible for the therapist's behavior.

Another source of some past ambivalence toward a colleague's sexual relationships with patients was psychiatry's attitude of tolerance of unconventional behavior. Psychiatrists are known to be at the more liberal end of the spectrum of medical specialists and to be more tolerant of deviance than, for example, are surgeons. This can lead to the characterization of a therapist's sexual relationship with a patient as "just" an affair or an aberration that needs to be approached by understanding the dynamics. Understanding is certainly appropriate; however, understanding alone can minimize the ethical and clinical violation.

Mounting experience has indicated that many of the abusing therapists have serious character problems and may not be easily treatable or rehabilitatable, although there does not appear to be one profile that characterizes all of them (Schoener et al. 1989). Although there is often more than one sexual relationship with patients, a single such relationship that takes place during a crisis in the therapist's life sometimes does occur. Although false accusations also exist, they are relatively rare (Benedek 1989). Most patients tell the truth about a history of sexual relations with a therapist. The power of the transference and the duration of its effects is a crucial aspect of the dynamics of the relationship that is increasingly recognized and acknowledged. The idea that the woman is a free participant in the relationship and that therefore it is one involving mutually consenting adults ignores this aspect.

REACTIONS OF THE INDIVIDUAL

The therapist who learns about a colleague's sexual relationship with a patient may react defensively to protect himself or herself against the feelings stirred up by this knowledge. This is one way to create some distance. It helps one to feel more protected and removed. The offending therapist can then be thought of as someone who belongs to an "other" group, with whom one does not identify. If the therapist is a respected person, the patient's accounts are too detailed to be dismissed, or there are too many reports to ignore, distancing is obviously more difficult. The very specific account by a patient, with convincing details may also break through the denial. Then there is a sense of betrayal, loss, disappointment, and disillusionment. It can be experienced as a loss of the colleague as well as of loss of regard for him.

Lymberis (1990) described the feelings of betrayal she had when she learned the details of a patient's previous sexual experience with a respected senior member of her psychiatric community. She also felt betrayed by the community that had tolerated his behavior and covered it over, and for a time she considered resigning from the group. This is not an isolated reaction. Another therapist described withdrawing from holding office in an organization in which an offending member had been active. This therapist was reluctant to continue to identify himself with the organization that had supported the other therapist.

It is also not uncommon to feel some anxiety about retaliation at the thought of taking action against a powerful member of the community who is reported to have had sexual relations with patients. The fantasy is that if someone with parental status has been able to violate boundaries, then is anyone safe? It can be a regressive experience, making the colleague feel like a child among powerful adults.

If the information becomes known in the community, other patients and students and colleagues become concerned. The other activities of this therapist are called into question, such as his teaching or referrals. If there is reason to doubt his judgment or integrity, it raises doubts about things that have no direct relationship to the sexual misconduct.

The therapist who knows about the sexual misconduct can feel isolated and lonely, especially if it is not publicly known and cannot be shared because of confidentiality. One's personal estimation of the abusing therapist has to be revised. The shift can involve a process akin to mourning, taking place over time and in a variety of contexts. Patients also describe how isolated they feel when they find themselves caught up in a relationship they feel is humiliating and degrading but cannot escape. It is possible for the subsequent therapist to feel identified with the patient and understand the patient's acquiescence and feel a similar conflict between taking action and remaining passive. This interplay of identification and distancing may be different for subsequent therapists, both male and female.

If others are reluctant to believe or respond appropriately to the information, it can paralyze the subsequent therapist, who needs collegial support to process this difficult situation. This may change with increasing publicity and recognition.

Another common reaction to hearing about patient-therapist sex is anger. The subsequent therapist can become very angry at the previous therapist. This anger can be displaced onto the patient who becomes the messenger of unwelcome information by confronting the new therapist.

For example, a therapist had seen a patient for a consultation because of distress resulting from sexual relations with another therapist whom the second therapist knew. The second therapist was outraged. He felt that he could not treat this patient unless she reported the sexual relationship to some authorities, and some punitive action could be initiated. The patient was reluctant to do this. The treatment was stalled and then interrupted. The second therapist's anger interfered with his being responsive to the patient and with his being able to treat her appropriately.

If a second therapist becomes preoccupied with bringing an abusing therapist to justice, this position can interfere with the capacity to help the patient with other aspects of her life and with the ability to do appropriate therapy, such as working toward understanding what the experience revived or the trauma of the encounter. The agenda of getting the first therapist punished interferes with mastery and resolution.

However, having the first therapist punished or his license removed may be important to the patient in countering her feelings of helplessness and victimization.

The second therapist can also feel helpless to do anything about the injustice or about the offending therapist and therefore about helping the patient. This confuses the treatment objectives with bringing the offending therapist to justice or redressing the wrong. Schoener (1990) described frequent mistakes made when working with victims of sexual misconduct by professionals. He included as mistakes the following: undue focus on the client filing a complaint, undue focus on the client's "anger," setting limits about one's "legal involvement," and bending rules for the client. The subsequent therapist may identify to some extent with the therapist who had the sexual relationship. One may become protective, particularly if one has had similar impulses, and look for ways of thinking about it that make it seem more acceptable or more tolerable. This can interfere with turning full attention to the patient's needs and with one's judgment about what is most helpful to the patient.

Attempts to deal with this can also lead to a primitive and global punitive attitude toward the offending therapist. Laws making sex between therapist and patient a criminal offense have been enacted in some states and proposed in others. However, some believe that the regulation or criminalization of the therapist's behavior is depreciating to the patient, who is not permitted to behave as a consenting adult. This applies particularly to relationships that begin some time after the treatment relationship is over. On the other side is the position that the transference lasts for a long time and always distorts the "free" choice of the patient or former patient. This distortion is perhaps never gone from the relationship.

DYNAMICS OF PATIENT-THERAPIST SEX FOR THE THERAPIST

Detailed knowledge about the dynamics of sexual involvement with patients is still being acquired. There have been some recent studies (Brodsky 1989; Gabbard 1989; Schoener et al. 1989) but none yet with depth or over a long period of time. It does appear that there is no one pattern that describes all situations. Data about the long range results of treatment programs, rehabilitative efforts, and educational approaches are also not yet available. It seems clear that this is not a problem to be solved by education alone, although there have been few explicit educational efforts within training programs up to the present.

A statement that it is unethical is not enough to prevent sex between therapists and patients. Some therapists become sexually involved with patients in the face of explicit ethical statements and rulings and take risks to their careers and personal relationships. Some have even served on ethics committees (e.g., of the American Medical Association and of the American Psychiatric Association). Twemlow and Gabbard (1989) and Brodsky (1989) reviewed some of the dynamics involved, noting that the therapeutic situation normally provides gratifications for the therapist as well as for the patient. They discussed the continuum of gratifications one derives from patients. Sexual and emotional fulfillment is at one extreme end; other more common rewards include the clinical data the patient provides for the therapist's education and career advancement and the expectable gratification one gets from doing a good job.

The abusing therapist is not necessarily manifestly disturbed. From their experience treating offending therapists and patients who have been abused, Twemlow and Gabbard (1989) found that many therapists who are engaged in boundary violations do not manifest sufficient psychological disturbance for this to be noticed by their colleagues. They divided sexually abusing therapists into three categories: the psychotic, the antisocial, and the "lovesick." They described the "lovesick" therapist as someone involved in a pathological falling-in-love process. This is an intense regressive dyadic relationship with little guilt. It is not with a whole person with whom there is a mutual relationship, but rather with part objects, and is a relationship where "only the idealized aspects of self and object exist" (p. 78). The authors maintained that behind the therapist's idea that he is giving the patient the love she did not receive in her early life or the omnipotent rescue fantasies that therapists sometimes have, there is an underlying destructive and sadistic nature to the relationship. They emphasized that these therapists have narcissistic problems and that an ego boundary disturbance is part of the lovesick state. They considered the lovesickness as a perversion because of the excitement that is associated with the risks taken and because of the sadistic nature of the underlying wishes.

Gabbard and Twemlow (1989) also considered the role of some patients in involving the therapist as part of an erotic transference or to avoid engaging in therapeutic work. A patient may attempt to involve a second therapist in the same way. They described a patient who thwarted the therapist's efforts to help her, insisting that the only way he could help was by a sexual relationship in which he would bring her to orgasm. He tried to give her an orgasm and failed, and then she did the same thing with another therapist.

Brodsky (1989) described the characteristics of offenders in interview studies of therapists from several disciplines and from a review of cases brought to ethics committees, licensing boards, and litigation. The abusing therapist in those studies was likely to be male, older than the patient, with some unsatisfactory love relationships in his own life. He often crossed other boundaries as well as sexual ones, such as being involved in business dealings with patients and talking to patients about details of his personal life. He was also likely to be an isolated professional and, more than other people, was likely to have had the experience of boundary violations with his own therapist. As further data accumulate, these profiles may change. Grandiosity—a sense of not being bound by rules—characterizes many abusing male therapists. Rescue fantasies appear to be important in the dynamics of some female therapists.

PSYCHOTHERAPY WITH PATIENTS WHO HAVE HAD SEX WITH PREVIOUS THERAPISTS

The subsequent therapy of patients who have had sexual relations with previous therapists is usually difficult, more difficult than the initial treatment (Apfel and Simon 1985). Not only are the original issues the patient brought to therapy unresolved, but there is the occurrence of the sexual acting. This also introduces the problem of the effects of a real trauma on the therapy.

The first goal is to establish trust. Many patients who have had sexual relations with therapists speak of the problem of reestablishing trust or developing trust with a new therapist. The patient may have to reject the next therapist, expressing the rage and disillusionment in relation to the previous therapist that were not expressed the first time. Patients are very sensitive to the style and attitudes of the subsequent therapist. A therapist who appears too detached, too intellectual, too remote, or too invested in his or her own agenda, can be rejected. An optimal response is a combination of empathy, a sense of distress or even outrage that this occurred, and the capacity to express this so that the patient feels it as genuine and at the same time feels safe to explore her own issues.

The problem of choosing the right therapeutic approach may seem insurmountable to the subsequent therapist. It is important to remember that the patient may need to find every approach unsatisfactory and be enraged at every subsequent therapist to some extent and for some time. The therapist needs to balance the willingness to be flexible with a consistent orientation not to enact but to understand. Although appropriate approaches vary, the one thing they all have in common is to contain a genuine response on the part of the subsequent therapist. The patient needs to feel that the therapist takes this experience seriously, is disturbed by it, is compassionate with the patient, does not blame her, and is prepared to deal with the issues that are aroused.

Assessing the past history is important. If the patient is in crisis, the therapist has the problem of obtaining the story and assessing its accuracy. Asking about details may appear judgmental to the patient. Apfel and Simon (1985) cited their experience that "stories of bizarre sexual practices with the previous therapist are . . . confirmatory of the tale rather than weakening its credibility" (p. 64). They stated that the importance of a nonjudgmental role in the attempt to help the patient integrate to the reality of her experience is greater than the need to establish the absolute veracity of the story.

If one judges the patient or devalues or blames her, empathy is difficult and this can also give rise to depression and helplessness in the therapist. In the situation described above in which the therapist heard about her patient's sexual experience after ECT, the second therapist shared the patient's sense of helplessness, which also represented a response to the patient's experience of finding it impossible to involve anyone in doing anything about the abusing therapist's behavior, even after she had complained. This feeling of helplessness was intolerable to the second therapist, who collaborated with the patient in not addressing the whole issue. Some years later, when publicity in the press about other individuals made it more acceptable to discuss the whole problem, the second therapist realized how harmful the silence had been to the patient, and how outraged she herself had felt.

PSYCHOTHERAPY OBJECTIVES

Beyond establishing trust and assessing the history, the psychotherapy objectives involve exploring the meaning of the experience and the patient's reactions in relation to her life circumstances and her psychopathology and working through all aspects of the experience that are important. This requires taking a sensitive and flexible approach, but also maintaining a therapeutic stance.

The decision about reporting can change in the course of therapy. The patient may for a time have no interest in reporting or taking legal action and then change her mind. She may be strongly invested in bringing the former therapist to justice. The current therapist needs to help the patient determine the implications of one or another course and to offer help without intruding his or her agenda. What course will be most helpful (and the patient's agenda) will vary from patient to patient. Decisions about reporting may come into conflict with a mandatory reporting regulation and this can pose a dilemma for the therapist: whether to give priority to the patient's confidentiality or the requirement for reporting. From a clinical point of view the patient's needs take priority. Schoener (1990) warned about the problems of not forewarning a patient about the limits of confidentiality and the clinician's mandatory reporting responsibility. He cited his own statement to clients in his clinic in Minnesota in which he told them that he might be obliged by law to report to an official body and cautioned clients not to reveal the identity of the former therapists initially until he had learned enough about the situation to know what the requirements were.

A common mistake made by subsequent therapists is to fail to recognize the positive feelings the patient may have toward the former therapist and the gains that may have been made in that treatment. Schoener (1990) pointed out that focusing on the positive feelings can support the patient's self-esteem and her understanding of why she stayed in the relationship or had difficulty sorting out what was going on. There can be a repetitive aspect to the therapy. The victim often needs to tell her story many times. The therapist must be able to tolerate hearing it and the associated affect. Marital, sexual, and family problems are not uncommon; sometimes these were the original presenting complaints in the first therapy. These are likely to have been intensified by the sexual relationship.

There are some parallels between working with a patient who has had sex with a therapist and work with other kinds of victims. Lion (1979) referred to two kinds of reactions when encountering victims of violent acts: 1) reaction formation and isolation and 2) anxiety and avoidance. He stated that if the victim can be seen as provocative, such as in the case of rape or wife battering, this makes it seem less likely that the violence will occur without provocation. One can maintain the illusion that one can protect oneself against this happening. This kind of mechanism has been reported concerning attitudes of lovers and family toward rape victims as well (Nadelson et al. 1982; Notman and Nadelson 1976). Conceptualizing the violence as an illness, such as in the studies of abused children where the abusers are sometimes described as mentally ill, also enables distance to be maintained (Lion 1979). Intellectualization diminishes the psychiatrist's or physician's anxiety. The idea that provocation, especially sexual provocation, "deserves" a primitive response has colored the approach to rape victims for many years. If the victim "asked for it," there then appears to be some justice in what happens to her. Blaming the victim of rape is accentuated by societal attitudes toward sexuality, in which women are held responsible for sexual transgressions (Notman and Nadelson 1982). These attitudes of blame extend to the patient who becomes sexually involved with her therapist.

As with rape victims, patients who have been sexually abused by therapists are likely to feel guilt and that they have some responsibility even if it is clearly stated that this is not so. They feel often that they lack credibility in stating their concerns. At the same time, it may be difficult for the patient to give up the idea that she was really the therapist's favorite patient or perhaps the only one with whom he had (or she had) a sexual relationship. Acknowledgment that this is not so, can bring a real sense of loss and disappointment. Sometimes this realization makes a patient willing to report the relationship or bring suit. It makes it clear to her that this was not a special friendship or love relationship. The absence of the "specialness" can also make subsequent therapy seem paler and not as gratifying.

A sensitive therapeutic issue is the role of the patient's past history in making her vulnerable to the abuse. This is important to work through, but it can also seem like blaming the patient if the subsequent therapist focuses on her readiness to acquiesce or even seek out such a relationship.

CONCLUSIONS

Learning about sexual boundary violations in a previous therapy creates an intrusion into a current treatment. It calls for some response to the real situation and for the capacity of the subsequent therapist to sort out his or her own countertransference responses from the needs of the patient. It is also important to gain an understanding of what might have brought about the violation without simplistically blaming the victim. In thinking about the offending therapist one must deal with anger, the mechanisms of denial and avoidance, and identification with the victim and, in some cases, the therapist.

Further experience will expand our knowledge as to when a therapist is rehabilitatable or treatable and when not and how best to work with the patients. Evaluating what is helpful and appropriate can be difficult. Sometimes assessing the nature of the trauma is complex because, although some situations are black and white, others are gray, such as social contact or touching under certain circumstances. Honesty and examination of one's own responses is important in the further therapeutic experience of the patient.

REFERENCES

American Psychological Association: Report of the task force on sex bias and sex role stereotyping in psychotherapeutic practice. Am Psychol 30:1169–1175, 1975

Apfel R, Simon B: Patient-therapist sexual contact, II: problems of subsequent psychotherapy. Psychother Psychosom 43:63–68, 1985

Benedek E: Forensic implications of false allegations of sexual abuse. Paper presented at the annual meeting of the American Psychiatric Association, San Francisco, CA, May 1989

Bouhoutsos J, Holroyd J, Lerman H, et al: Sexual intimacy between psychotherapists and patients. Professional Psychology: Research and Practice 14:185–196, 1983

Brodsky A: Sex between patient and therapist: psychology's data and response, in Sexual Exploitation in Professional Relationships. Edited by Gabbard G. Washington, DC, American Psychiatric Press, 1989, pp 15–25

Gabbard G (ed): Sexual Exploitation in Professional Relationships. Washington, DC, American Psychiatric Press, 1989

Gartrell N, Herman J, Olarte S, et al: Psychiatrist-patient sexual contact: results of a national survey. Am J Psychiatry 143:112–131, 1986

Holroyd JC, Brodsky A: Psychologists' attitudes and practices regarding erotic and nonerotic physician contact with patients. Am J Psychol 32:843–849, 1977

Kardener SH, Fuller M, Mensk IN: A survey of physicians' attitudes and practices regarding erotic and nonerotic contact with patients. Am J Psychiatry 130:1077–1081, 1973

Lion JR: Some emotional reactions associated with the study of victims. Paper presented at APA Task Force Symposium on Psychiatric Aspects of Terrorism, Baltimore, MD, September 1979

Lymberis M: Psychological aspects of therapist sexual abuse. Paper presented at a meeting of the Boston Psychoanalytic Society, Boston, MA, February 1990

Nadelson C, Notman M, Zackson H, et al: A follow-up study of rape victims. Am J Psychiatry 139:1266–1270, 1982

Notman M, Nadelson C: The rape victim: psychodynamic considerations. Am J Psychiatry 133:408–413, 1976

Perry J: Physicians' erotic and nonerotic physical involvement with patients. Am J Psychiatry 133:838–840, 1976

Pope KS, Bouhoutsos J: Sexual Intimacy Between Therapists and Patients. New York, Praeger, 1986

Pope KS, Levenson H, Schover LR: Sexual intimacy in psychology training: results and implications of a national survey. Am Psychol 34:682–689, 1979

Schoener GR: Frequent mistakes made when working with victims of sexual misconduct by professionals. The Minnesota Psychologist, pp 5–6, 1990

Schoener G, Milgrom J, Luepker E, et al: Psychotherapists' Sexual Involvement with Clients. Minneapolis, MN, Walk-In Counseling Center, 1989

Twemlow S, Gabbard G: The lovesick therapist, in Sexual Exploitation in Professional Relationships. Edited by Gabbard G. Washington, DC, American Psychiatric Press, 1989, pp 71–87

Concluding Reflections

John C. Nemiah, M.D.

The stock image of the psycho-therapist impassively and distantly, like some deistic god, viewing the gyrations of his patient's world lends itself to caricature but hardly to imitation. It is, indeed, an inherently false depiction of the therapist-patient relationship, for, as the word *relationship* implies, both therapist and patient share the deeply intimate and active goal of helping the patient resolve psychological conflicts that generate painful symptoms and distorted views of human interactions.

Seen from the outside, the therapeutic relationship often appears impersonal and one-sided. The patient tells all; the therapist reveals nothing of autobiographical facts or private values. But this is a surface calm only, for behind the seeming inactivity, the therapist's "evenly suspended attention" (as Freud [1912] called it) is engaged in an intensely active pursuit of an empathic understanding of the patient's inner life. This evenly suspended attention creates "for the doctor a counterpart to the 'fundamental rule of psychoanalysis' [i.e., free association] which is laid down for the patient. Just as the patient must relate everything that his self-observation can detect, and keep back all the logical and affective objections that seek to induce him to make a selection from among them, so the doctor must put himself in a position to make use of everything he is told for the purposes of interpretation and of recognizing the concealed unconscious material without substituting a censorship of his own for the selection that the patient has foregone. To put it in a formula: he must turn his own unconscious like a receptive organ towards the transmitting unconscious of the patient. [And thus] the doctor's unconscious is able, from the derivatives of the unconscious which are communicated to him, to reconstruct that unconscious, which has determined the patient's free associations" (Freud 1912, pp. 115–116).

Freud was, of course, focusing here on the central feature of one specific type of psychotherapy, namely psychoanalysis, and its derivative, psychodynamic insight psychotherapy. The psychotherapist is, however, often more visibly and intentionally active when patients need it—when, for example, they lack the capacity for engaging in insight psychotherapy, when they need active encouragement and support or require the setting of limits to potentially self-destructive behavior, or when the specific techniques of behavior therapy are indicated. And even in the purest form of insight psychotherapy, the absolute anonymity of the therapist is an ideal never completely achieved, because, as has often been pointed out, the way a therapist dresses and the decor of his or her office or the books displayed on the shelves all inevitably betray his or her incognito.

However that may be, most psychotherapists, whatever the form their treatment takes, attempt to keep their personal characteristics muted within the therapeutic relationship and to maintain the major focus on their patients' needs and clinical problems. And they try to provide their patients with a therapeutic environment that is steady, consistent, and free of unnecessary distortions—a cloister, so to speak, in which the work of treatment can go on without extraneous interruptions. More often than not, this ideal can be closely approximated, and the course of therapy is usually subjected to only minor dislocations.

But, as the chapters in this book amply demonstrate, the unexpected may happen, and personal crises in a therapist's life may threaten to tear the fabric of the therapeutic process. Serious illness (sometimes leading to death), pregnancy, a busy schedule in professional organization or public life activities—all of these may, in varying degrees, interrupt the even, regular flow of therapeutic hours. And even when the therapist is physically present for his or her patients, his or her mind and attention may be seriously distracted by grief over personal losses, by the anxieties resulting from stressful life events, or by a confounding countertransference aroused by a patient's problem that mirrors the therapist's own.

The phenomena described by the authors of this volume have been observed and studied by students of psychotherapy in only the most fragmentary fashion, and the literature concerning them is sparse. It is a merit of this book that it presents in detail and from the personal experiences of the authors the difficulties posed for the therapeutic process when real-life problems beset psychotherapists themselves. The reader may find the complexity and confusion of that detail daunting, and, indeed, it is hard at this point in our study of these problems to categorize or systematically classify the various disruptions in therapists' lives or to make valid generalizations about their effects on the course of therapy.

Some features are clear. Obviously, for example, the results of such disruptions will often be determined by the specific circumstances of individual cases. The needy, dependent patient in a supportive relationship may be more seriously disturbed by the actual absence of a sick therapist than by the psychological "absence" of a therapist who, though preoccupied with personal anxieties, maintains a regular schedule of hours. On the other hand, the process of insight psycho-therapy may be significantly hampered when personal anxieties dull the therapist's capacity for intuitive observation and interaction. In what the authors of this book have revealed for us about their personal experiences, the reader may find only a confusing, kaleidoscopic jumble. This is inevitable, given the complexity of the problems that occur when the harsh realities of the therapist's own world intrude on the therapeutic relationship. However, if a more precise categorization of these problems is not now possible, it is a useful initial approach to their understanding to see the universe of the problems as a whole. Our authors have opened the door on an aspect of psychotherapy that needs further study and elucidation.

Moreover, if categorization of the problems is difficult, their solution is even more elusive. Perhaps the first step in that direction is to allow ourselves to recognize that the problems exist. The paucity of literature concerning the various situations that our authors have described for us is mute evidence of the tendency of even skilled therapists to deny their existence. It is a tribute to our authors' openness that they have been willing to share with us the variety of difficulties they have en-countered. In courageously breaking the silence, they have not only allowed us to see the nature of the problems that potentially confront all of us as therapists, but they have made it easier for us to face them ourselves with equal insight and forthrightness. That is a hopeful be-ginning.

REFERENCE

Freud S: Recommendations to physicians practising in psycho-analysis (1912), in The Standard Edition of the Complete Psychological Works of Sigmund Freud, Vol 12. Edited and translated by Strachey J. London, Hogarth Press, 1958, pp 109–120

Index

*Page numbers printed in **boldface** type refer to tables or figures.*

Therapist (*continued*)
  social isolation of, in small
    community settings, 13–15
  supervision of. *See* Supervision
  vulnerability of, 47
 Therapy. *See* Psychotherapy
 Training, as reason for
 therapist's absence, 72
 Transference
 aging of therapist and, 53–54
 maternal, therapist's
   pregnancy and, 129
 patient's sexual encounter with
   therapist and, 166
 preceding therapy, in small
   community settings, 5

in psychoanalytic candidates,
  73
as reaction to therapist's illness
  or injury, 68–69
therapist's divorce and, 99
therapist's illness or injury and,
  30
therapist's losses and, 58–62
Transfer syndrome, 72
Trust, in therapy with patients
  who have had sexual
  encounters with a previous
  therapist, 167

Urban settings, small community
  settings versus, 2–3